Safeguarding Adults in Nursing Practice

Ruth Northway
and Robert Jenkins

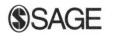 |

Los Angeles | London | New Delhi
Singapore | Washington DC

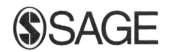 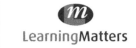

Learning Matters
An imprint of SAGE Publications Ltd
1 Oliver's Yard
55 City Road
London EC1Y 1SP

SAGE Publications Inc.
2455 Teller Road
Thousand Oaks, California 91320

SAGE Publications India Pvt Ltd
B 1/I 1 Mohan Cooperative Industrial Area
Mathura Road
New Delhi 110 044

SAGE Publications Asia-Pacific Pte Ltd
3 Church Street
#10–04 Samsung Hub
Singapore 049483

Development editor: Eleanor Rivers
Production controller: Chris Marke
Project manager: Diana Chambers
Copy editor: Sue Edwards
Marketing manager: Tamara Navaratnam
Cover design: Wendy Scott
Typeset by: Kelly Winter
Printed by: MPG Books Group, Bodmin, Cornwall

Library of Congress Control Number: 2012953311

British Library Cataloguing in Publication data

A catalogue record for this book is available from
the British Library

ISBN 0–978–1–4462–5637–4
ISBN 0–978–1–4462–5638–1 (pbk)

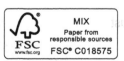

MIX
Paper from
responsible sources
FSC
www.fsc.org   FSC® C018575

Contents

Foreword

Safeguarding adults is a relatively new item on the nursing agenda. Safeguarding children from abuse has received more attention and prominence, and there are books available for nurses to understand this difficult area of care. More recently, a very bright light has been shone on the inadequate attention paid to safeguarding adults in care settings. Harrowing reports of abuse of adults, including older people, have been exposed and, while in the last decade policy frameworks and legislation to protect adults have been implemented, there is no textbook resource to advise and guide nurses in how they can handle these sensitive and complex issues.

Ruth Northway and Robert Jenkins have significant professional and personal knowledge and backgrounds in the care of people with learning disabilities. This includes an involvement in running courses concerning safeguarding for nurses across all fields of practice. They have used their expertise to create a book for the Transforming Nursing Practice series that addresses the shortfall in accessible reading for nurses in all fields in safeguarding principles. You will find in this book a wealth of information on the major issues around safeguarding adults as well as practical solutions to dealing with these issues in clinical settings, including interprofessional and interagency collaboration.

The authors' aim in this book is to raise awareness of the vulnerability of adults and to really understand what that means. The accessible style of the book helps you to make links between theory and practice, and to think carefully about achieving a balance between protection and empowerment. The policy and legislative background to safeguarding is explained in a manner that will give you confidence in your knowledge of patients' and clients' rights, and how your practice can be improved.

Take your time in reading this informative book – it will serve you well to improve your understanding of the policy, practice and research underpinning safeguarding, and consequently your important role as an advocate for and safeguarder of the people in your care.

Shirley Bach
Series Editor

About the authors

Ruth Northway is currently Professor of Learning Disability Nursing at the University of Glamorgan where she also heads the Unit for Development in Intellectual Disabilities, and is Visiting Professor in the School of Nursing Studies at the University of Ulster. She teaches across a number of undergraduate and postgraduate courses and is the award leader for the MSc Professional Practice (Vulnerable Persons). She has both teaching and research interests relating to safeguarding and has published in this field. She is a Fellow of the Royal College of Nursing and Editor of the *Journal of Intellectual Disabilities*.

Dr Robert Jenkins is Principal Lecturer at the University of Glamorgan. He teaches across a number of undergraduate and postgraduate courses, and is vulnerable person's module manager for the MSc Professional Practice (Vulnerable Persons). He has teaching, practice and research interests relating to safeguarding, particularly regarding people with learning disabilities, and has published widely in this area. He was recently part of a research study exploring the motivations of perpetrators of abuse.

Acknowledgements

To our practice colleagues for sharing their experiences and expertise. To the students attending our MSc modules for their willingness to engage in critical debate. Most importantly, to people who have been labelled 'vulnerable' by others and who have taught us what it is like to encounter abuse and neglect.

Introduction

Who is this book for?

This book is written for students of nursing who are developing knowledge and skills relating to safeguarding adults. Although primarily aimed at students, it will also be useful for qualified nurses, improving their practice and their role as mentors to students. Any health professional may find aspects of the book helpful for reviewing practice and planning improvements.

Why *Safeguarding Adults in Nursing Practice*?

Safeguarding people from harm is a key role for nurses and nursing. However, it is only relatively recently that the importance of this has been recognised in policies and legislation.

Requirements for nurse education

The Nursing and Midwifery Council (NMC, 2010c) has included in its *Standards for Pre-registration Nursing Education* reference to the need for all nurses to be able to identify when individuals are at risk and in need of additional support to protect them from abuse. This book aims to help you to achieve this standard and to meet your responsibilities in safeguarding adults at risk of harm.

Book structure

Chapter 1 aims to set the scene for this textbook by helping you to develop an understanding of the term 'nursing' in relation to safeguarding vulnerable people. It then explores how some nurses in the past have engaged in abusive and questionable practices. It will also require you to examine critically the extent to which such practices have been deemed abusive and to understand the relevance of this to modern-day nursing practice. A number of common themes will be highlighted and explored that have arisen from many of the past abuse inquiries. Finally, the issues discussed in this chapter can help you to examine your own personal values and attitudes in order for you to enhance the service you provide for people in your care.

Chapter 2 will essentially help you to explore some of the different meanings of vulnerability and why it may be viewed as a multidimensional concept. You will be encouraged to reflect on some of the vulnerability issues that impact on patients and clients with whom you have worked. You will also be encouraged to think about the implications for practice.

Chapter 3 introduces you to some key aspects of ethics and ethical practice. Emphasis will be placed on you to develop 'ethical sensitivity' in order for you to be able to respond in a moral manner to the vulnerability of patients and clients in practice. It will be suggested that, if you are to safeguard people from abuse and neglect, you must have an understanding of key ethical perspectives and principles, so that you can recognise when such principles are at risk of being ignored, and so that ethical principles can inform your decision making.

Chapter 4 provides you with the opportunity to examine different forms of abuse and neglect. You will be asked to consider why specific types of abuse may be viewed as more severe than others. Neglect, in particular, poses many challenges for professionals and services as it can often be difficult to detect. You will be encouraged to explore thresholds for abuse and why some nurses take action while others do nothing, often depending on a number of different factors. Finally, consideration is given to supporting and empowering survivors of abuse.

Chapter 5 will introduce you to the concept of safeguarding and some of the reasons for moving away from the term 'adult protection'. The broader nature of safeguarding will be explored in that it encompasses both a proactive and reactive approach to harm, abuse and neglect. The principles that underpin safeguarding will be examined and some implications of a safeguarding approach for the development of practice considered. A 'stepped' approach will be argued with a number of actions at individual, professional, organisational and societal levels being required. Responsibilities and interaction at each of these levels will be considered.

Chapter 6 introduces you to policy and legislation relevant to safeguarding. You will be required to consider a number of barriers to implementation as well as the importance of nurses having both knowledge of key legislation and an understanding of how to apply it in practice. As policy and legislation are constantly evolving, you will be made aware of sources of information that can be used to keep up to date.

Chapter 7 aims to give you an understanding of the importance of your professional duties in relation to safeguarding and protecting the public. Professional codes will be explored as well as the difficulties in raising concerns regarding abuse and poor practice. You will be encouraged to reflect on aspects of professional practice, such as confidentiality, as well as some practice examples. Finally, you will be required to consider strategies for practice development in areas such as clinical supervision and reflective practice.

Chapter 8 will explore why it is important for you to work with other professionals and agencies in order to safeguard vulnerable people. Working with others can pose difficulties and a number of factors will be examined that may impact negatively on an interprofessional approach. These factors will be around issues such as professional roles and responsibilities, communication, information sharing, and team and agency dynamics. Finally, consideration will be given to approaches that may support better interprofessional and interagency working.

Chapter 9 will introduce you to a number of key systems that form part of an overriding systems approach to safeguarding vulnerable people. Specific attention will be given to exploring three such systems: clinical governance, risk management, and health and safety. Case studies and scenarios will be used to help you understand how such systems interconnect and relate to each other to form part of a safeguarding system.

Finally, Chapter 10 aims to give you an understanding of the importance of evidence-based practice related to safeguarding. You will be introduced to the stages of evidence-based practice as well as a range of activities that should help you to relate various aspects of research findings to your current practice. The challenges in undertaking research in this area will be explored before suggestions for possible further research are put forward.

Requirements for the NMC *Standards for Pre-registration Nursing Education* and the Essential Skills Clusters

The Nursing and Midwifery Council (NMC) has established standards of competence to be met by applicants to different parts of the register, and these are the standards it considers necessary for safe and effective practice. In addition to the competencies, the NMC has set out specific skills that nursing students must be able to perform at various points of an education programme. These are known as Essential Skills Clusters (ESCs). This book is structured so that it will help you to understand and meet the competencies and ESCs required for entry to the NMC register. The relevant competencies and ESCs are presented at the start of each chapter so that you can clearly see which ones the chapter addresses.

This book includes the latest standards for 2010 onwards, taken from the *Standards for Pre-registration Nursing Education* (NMC, 2010c). For links to the pre-2010 standards, please visit the website for the book at **www.uk.sagepub.com/learningmatters/**.

Learning features

Learning from reading text is not always easy. Therefore, to provide variety and to assist with the development of independent learning skills and the application of theory to practice, this book contains activities, case studies, scenarios, further reading, useful websites and other materials to enable you to participate in your own learning. You will need to develop your own study skills and 'learn how to learn' to get the best from the material. The book cannot provide all the answers – but instead provides a framework for your learning.

The activities in the book will in particular help you to make sense of, and learn about, the material being presented. Some activities ask you to reflect on aspects of practice, or your experience of it, or the people or situations you encounter. *Reflection* is an essential skill in nursing, and it helps you to understand the world around you and often to identify how things might be improved. Other activities will help you develop key graduate skills such as your ability to *think critically* about a topic in order to challenge received wisdom, or your ability to *research a topic and find appropriate information and evidence*, and to be able to *make decisions* using that evidence in situations that are often difficult and time-pressured. Communication and working as part of a team are core to all nursing practice, and some activities will ask you to carry out *team working* or think about your *communication skills* to help develop these. Finally, as a registered nurse you will be expected to *lead and manage* your own team, case load or area of care, and so some activities focus on helping you build confidence in doing this.

All the activities require you to take a break from reading the text, think through the issues presented and carry out some independent study, possibly using the internet. Where appropriate, there are sample answers presented at the end of each chapter, and these will help you to understand more fully your own reflections and independent study. You will gain most from the activities if you try to complete them yourself before reading the suggested answers.

The authors of this book have utilised authentic case examples for most of the activities, and suggested possible answers and outcomes. In each case study, individual identities have been anonymised and modified. However, such exercises only allow for a snapshot of practice issues to be explored. If you are faced with similar complex situations, then you should always seek further advice from others such as mentors, clinical supervisors, managers, multidisciplinary team members, academics, trade unions, professional associations, solicitors, etc. In the past, the NMC offered professional advice but has recently stated that it will no longer provide a professional advice line and instead will focus on its core regulatory functions. You may wish to reflect on this new stance and provide feedback to the NMC.

Remember, academic study will always require independent work; attending lectures will never be enough to be successful on your programme, and these activities will help to deepen your knowledge and understanding of the issues under scrutiny and give you practice at working on your own.

You might want to think about completing these activities as part of your personal development plan (PDP) or portfolio. After completing the activity write it up in your PDP or portfolio in a section devoted to that particular skill, then look back over time to see how far you have developed. You can also do more of the activities for a key skill that you have identified a weakness in, which will help build your skill and confidence in this area.

There is a glossary of terms at the end of the book that provides an interpretation of some of the terminology in the context of the subject of the book. Glossary terms are in **bold** in the first instance that they appear.

All chapters have further reading and useful websites listed at the end, with notes to show you why we think they will be helpful to you. The websites will also help you to remain up to date with developments in this aspect of practice as awareness of key issues grows and policies develop.

We hope that you find this book helpful in developing your professional practice and that it challenges you to ensure you provide care and support that reduces the risk of vulnerability and promotes dignity, respect and a positive quality of life. Good luck with your studies!

Chapter 1
Safeguarding, vulnerability and abuse
Understanding the context

NMC Standards for Pre-registration Nursing Education

This chapter will address the following competencies:

Domain 1: Professional values

2. All nurses must practise in a holistic, non-judgmental, caring and sensitive manner that avoids assumptions; supports social inclusion; recognises and respects individual choice; and acknowledges diversity. Where necessary, they must challenge inequality, discrimination and exclusion from access to care.

Domain 3: Nursing practice and decision-making

1. All nurses must use up-to-date knowledge and evidence to assess, plan, deliver and evaluate care, communicate findings, influence change and promote health and best practice. They must make person-centred, evidence-based judgments and decisions, in partnership with others involved in the care process, to ensure high quality care. They must be able to recognise when the complexity of clinical decisions requires specialist knowledge and expertise, and consult or refer accordingly.

9. All nurses must be able to recognise when a person is at risk and in need of extra support and protection and take reasonable steps to protect them from abuse.

NMC Essential Skills Clusters

This chapter will address the following ESCs:

Cluster: Organisational aspects of care

11. People can trust the newly registered graduate nurse to safeguard children and adults from vulnerable situations and support and protect them from harm.

By the first progression point:

i. Acts within legal frameworks and local policies in relation to safeguarding adults and children who are in vulnerable situations.

By entry to the register:

ix. Supports people in asserting their human rights.

x. Challenges practices which do not safeguard those in need of support and protection.

> ## Chapter aims
>
> By the end of this chapter you will be able to:
>
> - identify the core values of nursing and safeguarding vulnerable people;
> - discuss the common themes that have emerged from historical abuse inquiries;
> - recognise the implications for nursing practice.

Introduction

The evidence is growing that vulnerable adults may be more at risk from abuse compared to the general population. Hardly a month goes by now without some abuse scandal making news on the television or in national newspapers. It often involves a range of vulnerable adults, but certain groups of people, such as older people or those with a learning disability or mental health need, make up a large proportion of cases. It may seem that this is a new development as we are often not made aware of past failings. However, the abuse of those deemed in need of additional support has been going on for thousands of years. Sadly, some of these abuses have been carried out by nurses, either intentionally, unintentionally or as part of an abusive culture of care.

Angels of death

In 1993, nurse Beverley Allitt was given 13 life sentences for the murder and abuse of children in her care while working at a hospital in Lincolnshire. In 2008, male nurse Colin Norris was given five life sentences for murdering older people in his care in Leeds hospitals during 2002. Both these serial killers will be required to serve a minimum of 30 years in prison for their crimes.

The two cases above are thankfully still very rare events, but they do illustrate the evil intents of some nurses who choose to abuse and murder vulnerable patients in their care. This chapter will help you to develop an understanding of the term 'nursing' and explore some of the abusive and questionable practices that have arisen from previous and recent failures in care. It will also require you to examine critically the extent to which such practices have been deemed abusive and to understand the relevance to modern-day nursing practice. A number of common themes will be highlighted and explored that have arisen from a number of abuse inquiries. Some useful recommendations made to address the shortcomings highlighted in abuse investigations, at inquiries and in the media will be presented. Nurses as perpetrators, witnesses and receivers of disclosures concerning abuse and neglect will be discussed. Finally, the issues discussed in this chapter will also help you to examine your own personal values and attitudes in order for you to enhance the service of people in your care.

Nursing vulnerable people

Before discussing safeguarding issues related to nursing it would be sensible to start off by exploring what we understand by the term 'nursing'. Nursing is a diverse and complex activity with many facets. The Royal College of Nursing (RCN) defines nursing as:

> *the use of clinical judgement in the provision of care to enable people to improve, maintain, or recover health, to cope with health problems, and to achieve the best possible quality of life, whatever their disease or disability, until death.*
> (2003a, p3)

The RCN acknowledged the limitation of a single definition and also included six defining characteristics that should be used in conjunction with each other to capture the full breadth of what it believes nursing entails (see Table 1.1).

Activity 1.1   *Critical thinking*

- Consider the above definition and the unique characteristics of nursing developed by the RCN. Can other professionals lay claim to some or all of the elements of nursing?
- Highlight some of the main features and values of nursing. Pay particular attention to the safeguarding role of nursing.

You may find some other ideas you have not thought of in the discussion below and in the outline answer at the end of the chapter.

The RCN recognised that many other professions may lay claim to particular aspects of nursing highlighted in both the core definition and characteristics. However, it points out that the uniqueness of nursing lies in the totality of all parts not just particular aspects. It is the combination of all the elements that gives nursing its distinctiveness and the definition expresses the common core of nursing, which remains constant (RCN, 2003a). The core definition has three key areas: the use of clinical judgement, concern for health and enhancing quality of life. This in itself sets nursing apart from other professions, although most health professionals would argue that they use clinical judgement in their practice. There is also an expectation that nurses need to empower individuals, which inevitably means that they do more than just concern themselves with physical aspects of care such as mobility. They also have to deal with families and communities and thus take on elements of a social dimension.

In terms of safeguarding, people need to feel safe and trust nurses with their health and well-being, particularly when they feel vulnerable (you will explore the issue of vulnerability in more detail in Chapter 2). When people are in need of care they should expect to be treated with dignity and respect by nurses (NMC, 2008a). They also expect to have support with a range of daily living activities if they are unable to do these things themselves. This support may involve assistance with feeding, bathing and dressing as well as having psychological needs being met. The level of support and personal care required varies between individuals. For example, a

Number	Characteristic	Defining features
1.	A particular purpose	• Promoting health, healing, growth and development. • Preventing disease, illness, injury and disability. • Minimising distress and suffering. • Maintaining the best possible quality of life until its end.
2.	A particular mode of intervention	• Empowering people, and helping them to achieve, maintain or recover independence. • Identification of nursing needs: therapeutic interventions and personal care; information, education, advice and advocacy; and physical, emotional and spiritual support.
3.	A particular domain	• People have unique responses to and experience of health, illness, frailty, disability and health-related life events in whatever environment or circumstances they find themselves.
4.	A particular focus	• Is on the whole person and his or her responses rather than a particular pathological condition.
5.	A particular value base	• Based on ethical values that respect the dignity, autonomy and uniqueness of all human beings, the privileged nurse–patient relationship, and the acceptance of personal accountability for decisions and actions.
6.	A commitment to partnership	• Work in partnership with patients, their relatives and other carers, and in collaboration with others as members of a multidisciplinary team.

Table 1.1 Defining characteristics of nursing (adapted from RCN, 2003a)

person with **dementia** or **multiple sclerosis** may be able to perform some self-care, such as brushing his or her teeth, but may need support with shopping. A person may be able to dress themselves one day but not the next. Essentially, some individuals may be able to live independently while others need support with everyday activities.

The level of support or nursing care provided may be dependent on the type of service provided. There are nursing care services that deal with predominantly health needs and there are social care services that deal with social needs or personal care. The more dependent the person is, the more likely he or she will be in need of some form of residential care. Residential care can be provided in a variety of settings, such as ordinary houses, group homes, hostels, warden-controlled complexes and small or large hospital-type services. Residential care services tend to be based on the nature of the client group. So we have residential services for older people and for people with mental health problems or learning disabilities. These can be provided by both health and social services.

Activity 1.2   *Critical thinking*

Consider the following brief pen pictures and identify some of the likely biological, psychological and social aspects of nursing and support needs of each person.

John Adams is a 38-year-old man who was involved in a serious road accident. He is currently in a coma, on life support, in the critical care unit of a local NHS Trust hospital.

Lily Evans is a 48-year-old woman who has not left her home for ten years due to panic attacks.

Jean Davies is a 72-year-old woman who has angina and emphysema. She is attached to a portable oxygen supply.

The above pen pictures illustrate that each patient requirement is unique but also that there may be some similar nursing and support needs. These differences and similarities can be seen in the outline answer at the end of the chapter.

Historical background to poor standards of care

The last thing people expect is to be abused by people who are being paid to care for them. There is nothing in the above definition and characteristics of nursing that suggests it is concerned with abusing people under nursing care. However, hospital inquiries and personal accounts have implicated professionals, including nurses, in abusing individuals in their care. Large residential facilities are not the sole domain of abuse as both Brown (1999) and Manthorpe (1999) argue that no settings, including small community homes or even a client's family home, are immune from the potential of abuse.

In the past groups of individuals such as those with learning disabilities or mental health problems were cared for initially in institutions called asylums, which were renamed hospitals when the NHS was formed in 1948. During the 1960s, institutional-type care was called into question by Goffman (1961), who undertook some of the earliest research into the life of institutionalised people with mental health problems in America. He described how some of the patients were socialised into developing institutionalised types of behaviour. The negative effects of such institutional process and setting took away some of the residents' personality, skills and choices. A type of 'institutional neurosis' develops in which patients become overly passive and dependent on those caring for them and do not challenge inhuman or degrading treatments. It must be remembered that there is great variation between institutions and not all residents are adversely affected by their processes.

In the UK, numerous hospital scandals of the early 1970s reinforced the view that hospital care was not a suitable provision for people with learning disabilities. The first of these took place in Ely Hospital in Cardiff (Committee of Inquiry, 1969) and was exposed by the *News of the World* newspaper. This scandal brought home to the nation the reality that nursing staff themselves could be guilty of abusing people in their care.

Subsequent major inquiries are highlighted in Box 1.1.

Box 1.1: How abuse of those with learning disabilities came to light

- **1969 Ely**: Initial complaints ignored until nursing assistant sent letter to national newspaper.
- **1971 Farleigh**: Initial complaints ignored until student nurse made allegations to police.
- **1972 Whittingham**: Initial complaints from student nurses suppressed until two senior managers made complaints.
- **1978 Normansfield**: Initial complaints ignored until strike by nurses protesting against the consultant psychiatrist.
- **1992 Ashworth**: Patient made initial allegations and then Channel 4 undertook documentary.
- **2006 Cornwall**: Mencap raised concerns and a Healthcare Commission investigation was undertaken.
- **2007 Sutton and Merton**: Chief executive of the NHS Trust requested Healthcare Commission to investigate concerns.
- **2011 Winterbourne**: Initial complaints by nurse whistle-blower ignored until BBC *Panorama* documentary.

These, and personal accounts of abuse to be found in books such as *Tongue Tied* (Deacon, 1982) and *The Politics in Mental Handicap* (Ryan and Thomas, 1987), suggested that nurses had engaged in abusive practices towards people with learning disabilities in their care. The Healthcare Commission (2006) joint investigation report into the provision of services for people with learning disabilities at Cornwall Partnership NHS highlights some of the abuses that took place (see Box 1.2).

> **Box 1.2: Healthcare Commission (2006) joint investigation findings**
>
> - One person spent 16 hours a day tied to a bed or wheelchair.
> - One man told investigators that he had never chosen any of the places he had lived in as an adult.
> - More than two-thirds of the sites visited placed unacceptable restrictions on people living there. For example, it was found that some internal and external doors were kept locked by staff.
> - In one home taps had been removed and, in another, light fittings had been taken out.
> - Poor record keeping prevented effective care from being provided.
> - There was little evidence of effective guidelines on handling challenging behaviour or adherence to treatment programmes.
> - Physical restraint was being used illegally.
> - There was excessive use of medication to control unacceptable behaviour.
> - In two of the three centres, there were no treatment plans for those residing there.

It was not only nurses who were engaging in abusive practices but also social care professionals. Evidence was emerging that **pindown** was being used to restrain young people and a number of abuses were being exposed in children's homes. The 1998 Longcare inquiry revealed that a social worker in charge of people with learning disabilities was regularly engaging in abusive practices, including raping some of the female residents. Residents were also financially and psychologically abused, neglected, kicked, drugged, given cold showers and forced to eat food outside. Pring's (2011) follow-up account of some of the survivors of the abuse that took place in Longcare reveals that the victims are still suffering. Encouragingly, in spite of the appalling cruelty, some of the survivors demonstrated remarkable **resilience** and had the courage to help bring the abuser to justice.

It is not only people with learning disabilities who have suffered decades of abuse at the hands of professionals. There are similar abuse scandals in the fields of mental health and older persons' care. In 2002, the Commission for Health Improvement (CHI) investigated allegations of abuse of older people with mental health problems by care staff at Rowan Ward (Manchester Mental Health and Social Care Trust). The Commission generally focused on 'institutional-type abuse' rather than specific cases. Such abuses were found to be a lack of person-centred care, overuse of medication, lack of activities, lack of service user voice, poor living conditions and outdated nursing practices. It is not only public inquiries that bring abuse scandals to the attention of the public, but personal accounts and reports of institutional practices. Two such accounts that highlighted the poor standards of care of older people were published during the 1960s. Peter Townsend's *The Last Refuge* (1962) and Barbara Robb's report *Sans Everything* (1967) laid bare some of the questionable treatment of older people in the UK. Robb provided a report on behalf of an organisation that was concerned about the care of older people in the public sector. She compiled numerous accounts from nurses and social workers of appalling cruelty towards older people, many of whom had additional mental health needs. Such accounts included being denied basic necessities such as dentures, hearing aids and glasses, being left to remain idle and lonely, and generally being treated as if they were somehow less than human.

There is a suggestion that people who live in residential care cannot manage their lives in the same way as other people living in the community (Oliver and Barnes, 1998). However, not everyone shares these views and Jack (1998) questions much of the negative anti-residential care claims on the grounds that much of the work is biased and because institutions are wide and varied in nature. He feels that institutions involved in welfare provision all have the potential for the personal growth of the people within them. This is supported by groups such as My Home Life, a national movement aimed at improving the quality of life of those who are living in care homes for older people (for more information, see the website at end of this chapter). However, even Jack acknowledges that institutions have the potential to depersonalise individuals.

Recent reports and inquiries

The BBC *Panorama* current affairs programme in the early part of 2011 made a documentary about abuse at Winterbourne View, a private hospital for people with learning disabilities. An undercover reporter secretly filmed widespread abuse of the residents by a number of care staff. The film showed patients being pinned down, slapped, doused in water, verbally abused and taunted at the home. Shortly afterwards the company closed the home. The Care Quality Commission (CQC) found that Castlebeck Care had demonstrated systematic failure in ensuring residents living at the home were protected from risk and that staff did not understand the needs of the people for whom they were caring. The company had also failed to inform the CQC of serious injuries to some of the residents and that some of the residents had also gone missing. Eleven members of staff were convicted of abusing vulnerable adults in their care a year later in 2012. This case will be referred to in a number of subsequent chapters.

Activity 1.3   *Critical thinking*

Access the following link to witness the secret filming of the alleged abuse that took place at Winterbourne View in 2011: www.bbc.co.uk/programmes/b011pwt6. You may need some emotional support as some of the scenes are very distressing.

After viewing the film answer the following questions.

* What are your overall impressions?
* What types of abuse took place?
* Why did it need an undercover reporter to expose the abuse?
* How did the other residents who were not being abused react?

Read the following text for more information about this case.

You would probably have been very disturbed by the scenes that were filmed in this private hospital. However, some of these were similar to earlier abuses reported by investigative reporter Donal Macintyre in 1999 and 2003. He exposed similar abuses and neglect in residential care homes for older people and people with learning disabilities. They were also closed down after the abuses came to light. The type of abuse that caused most concern in the Winterbourne case was physical abuse. This type of abuse usually makes for a big headline or impact compared to neglect. The reasons for this will be explored in more detail in Chapter 4. Sadly, the reasons that undercover reporters have had to expose the abuse at some residential units are because often 'closed' cultures have developed in these places. The units tend to be isolated; the unit in Winterbourne was a first-floor area with restricted access. There was also a lack of external monitoring and appraisal by individuals not employed by the company. The lack of a reaction by some of the residents, who were not being abused at the time, was probably the most telling. Were they so used to seeing the staff behave in such a fashion that they were past caring? Were they so afraid of daring to show any emotion for fear they would be subjected to the abuse? These are, of course, just a couple of perspectives and, as the area of abuse is such a complex issue, there would be many more differing perspectives regarding the abuse that took place in this hospital.

It is not only large, long-term residential establishments that abuse occurs in. The National Health Service (NHS) has had a long history of inquiries into poor care practices and abuses on patients in its care. People with learning disabilities have above-average health needs compared to the general population (Backer et al., 2009; RCN, 2011). The NHS was founded on the principle of providing healthcare to all members of society based on need, including people with learning disabilities. Indeed, the famous quote by Aneurin Bevan, the founder of the NHS, *No longer will wealth be an advantage or poverty a disadvantage. Healthcare will be provided free of charge based on clinical need and not on ability to pay*, typifies the commitment of the NHS to disadvantaged people. However, a number of reports and recent inquiries into the premature deaths of people with learning disabilities support the view that this group of people are dying prematurely due to the indifference and neglect of healthcare professionals, including nurses.

The Disability Rights Commission (2006) found in its research that, as a group, people with learning disabilities were likely to die younger and suffer more from a number of conditions, particularly obesity and respiratory disease, as well as having fewer health investigations and screenings. The Commission also found that people with mental health problems are much more likely to have major health problems in areas such as obesity, smoking, heart disease, high blood pressure, respiratory disease, diabetes and stroke. One of the most worrying aspects of the report was that both groups of vulnerable clients may even have higher levels of ill health than was noted in their health records. It was felt that there were instances of **diagnostic over-shadowing**, in which the symptoms of ill health are thought to be a part of the mental health or learning disability condition and so are not investigated or treated.

The Mencap (2007) report *Death by Indifference* focused on institutional **discrimination** within the NHS against people with learning disabilities. It highlighted that appalling treatment of people with learning disabilities by professionals working in hospitals throughout the country had come to light. Its earlier report and campaign *Treat Me Right* (Mencap, 2004) exposed the unequal treatment that people with learning disabilities often experience from professionals working in healthcare. Partly in response to the growing evidence and findings from various reports, the Royal College of Nursing (RCN, 2011) has produced a useful guidance document for nursing staff on meeting the healthcare needs of people with learning disabilities. An independent public inquiry (Michaels, 2008) investigated access difficulties experienced by people with learning disabilities, including the six premature deaths of people with learning disabilities highlighted in the *Death by Indifference* report. This report from the inquiry made a number of recommendations in which, in order to improve matters such as compliance with the law, consulting both carers and clients, and improving data collection methods, all professionals must undergo training in learning disabilities, awareness raising and improved monitoring of health services. Sadly, there has been little significant improvement, five years on, with the aptly named progress report by Mencap (2012) *Death by Indifference: 74 deaths and counting.*

Similar issues are faced by older people within the NHS. The Older People's Commissioner for Wales (2012) is currently reviewing the hospital experiences of older people with regard to dignity and respect. What she has found to date is that the treatment of older people is shamefully inadequate. Many older people had low expectations regarding their care in hospital and the two main issues that came up time and time again were those of dignity and respect. This is why many, although not all, universities ensure that all student nurses have a placement with vulnerable groups of people such as older people and those with learning disabilities and mental health problems. The NMC also acknowledges this and encourages the involvement of service users in the training of nurses. *The Code: Standards of conduct, performance and ethics for nurses and midwives* (NMC, 2008a) clearly stresses that registered nurses *must* **advocate** on behalf of people in their care, helping them to access relevant health and social care, information and support. In order to do this, nurses should have an understanding of the needs of each of the client groups in their care.

Case study: A lack of dignity and respect

Mr Elfed Jones is an 80-year-old man who has been on a high-dependency ward of his local general hospital after a stroke. He has a slight speech impediment and has paralysis on his left side. His only living relative is his daughter who lives away and can only visit him at weekends. Mr Jones is a very private person and is very guarded regarding giving out his personal information. He does not like speaking on the ward as he can hear personal information being discussed around the bedside of other patients. He sometimes misses meals when he has to go for other treatments off the ward. He has complained to his named nurse, but she is seldom on the ward at the moment as she is undertaking further training. The staffing levels on the ward seem very low and often Mr Jones has to wait for long periods for a nurse to bring him a commode, which is not always clean. When he tries to speak to nurses they often finish his sentence for him, which makes him very angry. He has overheard a nurse referring to him as the moaning stroke patient in bed 4.

In the above case study it can be seen that there is very little dignity and respect shown to Mr Jones. At an organisational level, low staffing levels may indicate that this ward and its patients are not a priority. The lack of privacy may further reinforce this belief. Strangely, this can be seen with the pulling of curtains around a patient's bed in the belief that it respects the patient's privacy. There is an effort to respect privacy in that patients cannot see each other, but all the discussion can be heard by those in the vicinity. This would be of particular importance to Mr Jones as nurses caring for him should be aware of his sensitivity towards others 'knowing his business'. This may increase a patient's feeling of vulnerability and that he or she is not respected. The missing of meals may be yet a further example that patients are not afforded the dignity and respect they deserve. The most telling factors that would indicate that the nursing staff have shown little respect or dignity towards Mr Jones, are those of expecting him to use a dirty commode and referring to him as 'the moaning stroke patient in bed 4'.

Activity 1.4	Reflection

- Imagine yourself in Mr Jones's situation. How would you react?
- Remembering the effects that a stroke would have, would you feel able to voice your concerns?
- How would you feel if someone finished your sentences, was seldom available, made you wait for a long period for a commode, eventually gave you a dirty commode, and then referred to you in such a hurtful way?

You would probably experience a range of emotions and most people would not expect to be on the receiving end of this type of care. An outline answer is given at the end of the chapter.

It is not only people with learning disabilities, older people and those with mental health problems who receive questionable care from the NHS. An independent inquiry into care provided by Mid Staffordshire NHS Foundation Trust between January 2005 and March 2009, chaired by Robert Francis QC, was published in two volumes in 2010. It found poor and neglectful care in a number of areas such as nutrition and hydration, pressure area care, personal and oral hygiene, patient safety, continence and bladder and bowel care, cleanliness and infection control, privacy and dignity, diagnosis and treatment, communication and discharge management. The whole patient experience was very poor due to a culture within the Trust that did not provide good care for patients or a supportive working environment for staff. There was also evidence found of poor record keeping and bullying of staff, and one of the most concerning aspects of the inquiry was that some senior managers felt that there was nothing seriously wrong with the care provided by the Trust during this period.

For full details, access the following website for volume 1 at www.midstaffsinquiry.com/assets/docs/Inquiry_Report-Vol1.pdf; and for volume 2 at www.midstaffsinquiry.com/assets/docs/Inquiry_Report-Vol2.pdf.

Common themes emerging from abuse inquiries

There have been many inquiries and reports published over the years examining the causes of institutional abuse and offering some direction in preventing further abuses. Reder and Duncan make a radical proposal by stating that:

Since the findings of any next inquiry could reasonably be predicted before it has taken place, we would like to propose that no further inquiries are commissioned before all the training and resource deficiencies identified over the last thirty years have been remedied.
(2004, p95)

Many professionals involved in safeguarding share these views as common themes emerge from inquiries into institutional abuse. Therefore we know enough about the causes and we should know how to address each of the issues to ensure abuse is less likely to occur. A number of literature reviews and guidance on environments and cultures that promote abuse (Wardhaugh and Wilding 1998; Walshe, 2003; White et al., 2003; Royal College of Psychiatrists, 2004; Marsland et al., 2007; Aylett, 2008; Benbow, 2008) highlight some common themes (see Figure 1.1).

First, concerns are usually raised within the institution by some of the care staff witnessing abuse taking place. However, if these concerns are not dealt with appropriately, further concerns are usually made from outside the organisation by professionals, family/carers or service user groups. It is at this early stage that organisations should address staff concerns and deal with the issues

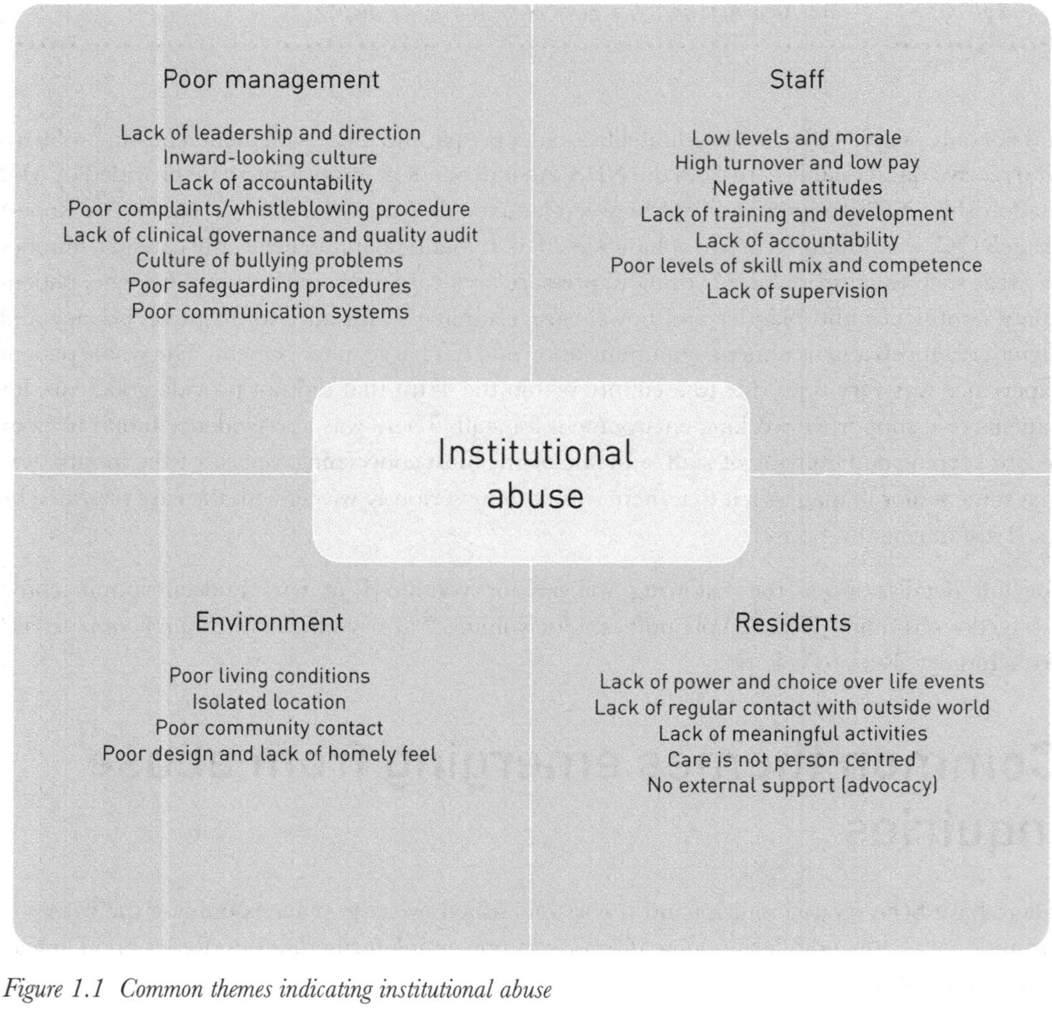

Poor management

Lack of leadership and direction
Inward-looking culture
Lack of accountability
Poor complaints/whistleblowing procedure
Lack of clinical governance and quality audit
Culture of bullying problems
Poor safeguarding procedures
Poor communication systems

Staff

Low levels and morale
High turnover and low pay
Negative attitudes
Lack of training and development
Lack of accountability
Poor levels of skill mix and competence
Lack of supervision

Institutional abuse

Environment

Poor living conditions
Isolated location
Poor community contact
Poor design and lack of homely feel

Residents

Lack of power and choice over life events
Lack of regular contact with outside world
Lack of meaningful activities
Care is not person centred
No external support (advocacy)

Figure 1.1 Common themes indicating institutional abuse

in a timely and effective manner. Organisations can send out a clear message that a zero tolerance towards any form of abuse is in operation. However, lessons from numerous inquiries clearly show that organisations fail to do this, and see abuse flourishing in various forms that often escalate into major problems.

The difficulty with institutional abuse is that it tends to remove responsibility for abuse away from individual practitioners. People can claim that 'it was not me but the system that was at fault'. For example, they could claim that it was common practice to shout at patients, allow them to miss meals or over-sedate them. However, nurses and other professionals contribute to the formation of the 'care culture' within their place of work. Nurses may feel that they are 'doing the best they can' in difficult environments and may feel powerless to influence wider cultural factors that lead to a corruption of care (Wardhaugh and Wilding, 1998). This feeling of powerlessness has been seen in past inquiries into abuse. It is therefore surprising to still see this and other themes reappearing in more recent exposés such as those of Rowan Ward, Longcare and Winterbourne (misuse and abuse of power, under-resourcing, poor complaints procedure, lack of training and staff support, inward-looking organisational culture and widespread apathy). It would seem that recommendations made in official inquiries are largely ignored or not implemented adequately. There may have been too much focus on getting rid of 'bad apples' in a quick fix strategy rather than taking a more measured response in dealing with wider institutional abuse and responsibility at all levels (Manthorpe and Stanley, 1999).

With regard to poor practice and abuse in the NHS, the Older People's Commissioner for Wales (2010) has made 12 recommendations to change the culture of caring for older people in Welsh hospitals (see Box 1.3). The main aim of these recommendations is to improve the dignity and respect shown to older people. These recommendations could equally be applied to the rest of the UK.

Box 1.3: The Older People's Commissioner for Wales (2010) recommendations to change the culture of caring for older people in Welsh hospitals

1. Stronger ward leadership is needed to foster a culture of dignity and respect.
2. Better knowledge of the needs of older people with dementia is needed, together with improved communication, training, support and standards of care.
3. Lack of timely response to continence needs was widely reported and is unacceptable.
4. The sharing of patients' personal information in the hearing of others should cease wherever possible.
5. Too many older people are still not being discharged in an effective and timely manner, and this needs urgent attention.
6. The appropriate use of volunteers in hospitals needs further development, learning from successful initiatives.
7. Staffing levels have to reflect the needs of older people both now and in the future.
8. Simple and responsive changes to the ward environment can make a big difference.

9. Effective communication can raise patients' expectations and involvement, and can improve their hospital experience.
10. The experience of older patients, their families and carers should be captured more effectively and used to drive improvements in care.
11. Good practice should be better identified, evaluated and learnt from to bring about improvements in care.
12. All those working with older people in hospitals in Wales should have appropriate levels of knowledge and skill.

Activity 1.5   *Critical thinking*

Consider the recommendations in Box 1.3 and select three that you feel could be addressed by your local hospital, for instance numbers 1, 2 and 8. Outline how hospitals could improve matters in each of these areas.

The following discussion offers some solutions that your local hospital may use in order to change to a more patient-focused culture. Further guidance is offered in the outline answer at the end of the chapter.

Recommendation 1 is probably the key to developing a culture of dignity and respect towards older people in the ward environment. The culture of an environment is often a reflection of the personality of the person in charge. Managers must have the necessary authority and skills of a strong leader to bring about change. They should have the opportunity to select their own staff teams and ensure that they have the necessary skills, knowledge and, most importantly, attitudes to foster a suitable culture. Managers should ensure that they regularly supervise, appraise and performance manage their staff.

Recommendation 2 is in response to the growing numbers of people who are likely to develop dementia in future years. It has been estimated that there will be 1.4 million people with dementia in the UK by the year 2038, with an expected cost of over £5 billion (DH, 2009a). The National Dementia Strategy (DH, 2009a) aims to improve the quality of life of people with dementia by addressing three main areas. The first is to reduce the **stigma** of having the label 'dementia' by ensuring people are better informed about the condition. The second is to ensure early diagnosis, support and treatment for people with dementia and their carers. The final area is to develop services in order to meet the changing care needs of individuals with dementia through a multidisciplinary team approach. It is therefore important for ward staff to have regular up-to-date training in dementia care.

Finally, recommendation 8 is concerned with listening to the people in your care. It is often the simple changes that can make the biggest differences to people's lives. Many patients complain about the visiting times for relatives. Visiting times should be flexible and responsive to patient need rather than the routine of the ward. It can be distressing to keep to patients' and relatives' established visiting times, for example insisting that relatives leave at certain times even when patients are clearly distressed at the time and need comforting. If wards have to keep to certain schedules, the reasons why should be clearly explained to relatives and patients. The siting and availability of phones should again meet the needs of older people. For example, they may need large-sized number pads on the phones as well as some privacy when using them. The point is that patients should be consulted when changes to ward environments and routines are planned.

Concern about the poor treatment of older people in health and social care settings is not just confined to Wales. A national organisation called Dignity in Care was set up in 2006 to address the situation. It also aims to put dignity and respect at the heart of all care services with a ten-point challenge.

1. Have a zero tolerance of all forms of abuse.
2. Support people with the same respect you would want for yourself or a member of your family.
3. Treat each person as an individual by offering a personalised service.
4. Enable people to maintain the maximum possible level of independence, choice and control.
5. Listen and support people to express their needs and wants.
6. Respect people's right to privacy.
7. Ensure people feel able to complain without fear of retribution.
8. Engage with family members and carers as care partners.
9. Assist people to maintain confidence and a positive self-esteem.
10. Act to alleviate people's loneliness and isolation.

The next section will consider nurses as perpetrators, witnesses and receivers of disclosures concerning abuse and neglect.

Nurses as perpetrators, witnesses and receivers of disclosures concerning abuse and neglect

As can be seen from the above discussions on institutional abuse, nurses have been perpetrators of abuse. Indeed, Davies and Jenkins state that:

> *It is evident in the professional arena that abuse of vulnerable people takes place in a variety of different settings perpetrated by a variety of different people who may belong to a variety of different professions or organisations.*
> (2004, p33)

However, very little research has been undertaken to understand why nurses and others engage in abusive practices. Some recent research by Davies et al. (2011) has sought to address this by exploring the **motivations** of perpetrators of abuse. They focused on two types of abuser.

- **The reactive abuser** – A demotivated, stressed and undervalued employee/family member who is poorly supervised and who abuses out of desperation due to impossible odds. Often this abuse is linked to a 'critical incident', where the potential perpetrator felt pushed to take the step towards becoming an abuser. For example, the employee felt pushed to react to an incident because he or she felt that nobody cared or listened.

- **The proactive abuser** – A 'bad apple' or serial abuser who actively seeks out vulnerable people by developing friendships or by working in caring in order to carry out acts of abuse. He or she can also create or take advantage of opportunities in which to abuse others. For example, the abuser offers to cover for a colleague knowing full well that the service is short-staffed and he or she will be able to work alone with a vulnerable adult for a short period of time. The abuser knows he or she will not be monitored and will be in the manager's good books because of volunteering to help out. The person may not abuse on the first occasion but will use it as a way of developing the relationship in order to abuse.

Davies et al. (2011) found that a diversity of motivations for the abuse of vulnerable adults was evident, some of which could be placed in the categories of proactive and reactive motivations. However, they found a third cluster of motivations that are more relational.

- **The relational abuser** – This type of abuse is when the abuser is related to the victim of abuse (son or daughter) and the motivations were more complex. For example, a son would abuse his father because he felt his father used too much physical force towards him when he was a child. He may also have felt that he did not live up to his father's expectations and was made to feel a failure. In this type of situation the abuser may believe that he or she is paying a parent back for the punishment received in childhood. This type of abuse may give support to the view that the abused go on to become abusers. While there may be some sympathy for the abuser in these types of situations because of the relationship, such abuse cannot be allowed to continue or not be investigated. Remember, as a nurse you are not the judge and jury, and this is best left to the legal system. In some of the cases in Davies et al.'s (2011) study, the parents just wanted the abuse to stop and were reluctant to help the police secure a prosecution.

Motivations were found rarely to occur in isolation and several issues within a category or between categories were found to be relevant in a single case. In terms of repeat offending, motivations tended to shift over time. (A case study in Chapter 9 will explore the reactive type abuser in more detail.)

Activity 1.6   *Critical thinking*

In terms of preventing abuse, what strategies could be employed to prevent each type of abuser outlined above engaging in abuse in a healthcare setting?

An outline answer is given at the end of the chapter.

The NMC (2002, p4) takes a clear stance on abuse with the statement that *zero tolerance of abuse is the only philosophy consistent with protecting the public*. The problem with this clear and commendable statement is that it does not give guidance to the nurse in interpreting how zero tolerance can be achieved as a professional duty. Davies and Jenkins argue that attempts to present guidance to nurses fall under three broad categories:

- *how the practice of an individual nurse is such that abuse is prevented;*
- *how the nurse holds a unique position in detecting and responding to abuse should it arise;*
- *how the nurse contributes to the development of a zero tolerance culture.*

(2004, p34)

Unfortunately, clarity on these three elements of nurses' responsibility in all situations would be impossible from a professional body. The responsibility of the nurse is defined in the NMC *Code* (2008a, p1). It clearly states that, as a registered nurse, the people you care for must be able to trust you with their health and well-being, and that you are personally accountable for actions and omissions in your practice.

To justify that trust, it further states that you must:

- *make the care of people your first concern, treating them as individuals and respecting their dignity;*
- *work with others to protect and promote the health and wellbeing of those in your care, their families and carers, and the wider community;*
- *provide a high standard of practice and care at all times;*
- *be open and honest, act with integrity and uphold the reputation of your profession.*

(NMC, 2008a, p2)

The nature of the above statements should be viewed as empowering as it encourages the nurse to rise above either a culture or specific individuals whose practice could be viewed as abusive. In accepting their own accountability, nurses will look for guidance from their professional body, the NMC, for more detailed advice. However, while the NMC *Code* offers general guidance on the behaviour and responsibility of the nurse, most of the guidance on the prevention, detection and management of abuse was contained in the document *Practitioner–Client Relationships and the Prevention of Abuse* (NMC, 2002). However, this document is no longer available and has been replaced with some guidance on general safeguarding issues. The NMC (2010a) defines safeguarding as:

a range of activity aimed at upholding a person's fundamental right to be safe. It means protecting patients and their families from all forms of harm, abuse and neglect, including poor practice.

It would seem that the NMC does not distinguish poor practice from abuse with regard to safeguarding people in the care of a nurse and this will be explored in more detail in Chapters 4 and 5. In spite of the above, it is therefore surprising that, when abuse is reported, it is usually by a single individual who has persisted with his or her claims – a single whistle-blower. In nursing there are a number of notable whistle-blowers who have been resolute in pursuing their allegations of abuse. The first was Graham Pink in 1990, when he highlighted poor care practices for older people in a hospital in Stockport by writing to *The Guardian* newspaper. Margaret Haywood filmed undercover for the BBC current affairs programme *Panorama*, to highlight the neglect of older people in a hospital in Sussex. The most recent nurse is Terry Bryan, who reported incidents to managers at Winterbourne View and to the Care Quality Commission, but little action was taken until *Panorama* broke the story. Surprisingly, the first two nurses were both struck off the professional register as a result of their whistle-blowing activities. This issue will be addressed in more detail in Chapter 7.

In the cases highlighted above, why do you think that some nurses will report abuse while others do not, particularly when they are both working in the same environments, under the same conditions and with the same patients and staff?

The following discussion will offer some reasons why nurses may be reluctant to report abuse, so there is no outline answer at the end of the chapter.

Implications for practice

People have different standards, thresholds, perceptions and values and therefore we sadly see that some people will not report abuse, when clearly it is very evident that it is taking place before their very eyes. The NMC is clear in that nurses are duty bound by their *Code* to *report concerns in writing if problems in the environment of care are putting people at risk* (2008a, p5). However, if you do not see it or believe it is abuse, you are unlikely to report it. Some individuals may fear the person who is committing abuse or may be being threatened by him or her. Some may believe that certain types of abuse such as neglect are not as serious as sexual abuse, so may wait a while in the hope it will not continue. Student nurses may want a good clinical report and feel that they should wait to report it later when they have left the environment. This 'wait and see' attitude is not unusual but should be viewed as accepting what is going on. Again, the NMC (2008a, p5) stresses that *you must act without delay if you, a colleague or anyone else may be putting someone at risk.*

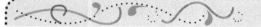

Chapter summary

Reading this chapter may have been very depressing for you as it has highlighted instances of abuse perpetrated by nurses. Fortunately, it must be remembered that the vast majority of nurses adopt the positive values and standards of nursing, and are a credit to the profession. It is also pleasing that many of the old institutions that were used to care for vulnerable groups are no longer here, and have been replaced with more modern and suitable services that have adopted person-centred approaches. Finally, it should be remembered that environments do not actually abuse patients/clients, although some types may make it more likely to happen; it is only people who abuse people. Therefore, nurses should remain vigilant at all times and report those who do.

Activities: Brief outline answers

Activity 1.1 Critical thinking, page 7

Most professional groups can claim some if not all of the main features and values of nursing highlighted below. However, the uniqueness of nursing is that the totality of caring is done by this one professional. The empowering, supporting and caring roles are central to nursing. The roles of other professionals and interprofessional working are explored in more detail in Chapter 8. In terms of safeguarding, we can see this is as an implicit and developing role of nursing.

Some of the main features and core values of nursing are that nurses should:

* demonstrate dignity and respect for those in their care;
* take a holistic view of caring for people and their carers;
* be person centred;
* safeguard clients' interests and protect them from harm;
* enhance clients' quality of life – at the very least should not make it worse;
* advocate on behalf of the client if he or she is being abused;
* empower individuals to protect themselves.

Activity 1.2 Critical thinking, page 9

Following are some of the likely support needs of the individuals concerned.

John Adams: He will be totally dependent on medical and nursing staff for all his biological needs. His psychosocial needs would be best met once he regains consciousness.

Lily Evans: She is likely to be self-caring so can wash, dress and feed herself. Her nursing support needs will centre on psychological aspects such as supporting her through her anxiety. Focus could also be put on maintaining and developing her friendships.

Jean Davies: She is likely to need support in caring for herself such as dressing, feeding, shopping etc. The oxygen will obviously create practical problems with these activities and she will need reassurance when she has difficulty with breathing and pain with her angina. The important thing is for her to try to maintain her social networks. When people develop disabilities, like Lily and Jean, their social networks tend to diminish.

Activity 1.4 Reflection, page 15

It may be very difficult to put yourself into the shoes of an older person if you are a younger person. However, you would probably be annoyed if other people always finished your sentences for you. You would probably feel even more upset at waiting for a long period to go to the toilet and would be horrified if the commode was dirty from the last person to use it. You may feel some sympathy towards the nursing staff as they always seemed short-staffed and consequently very busy. However, referring to you in such a derogatory term as well as not ensuring you had adequate nutrition would probably make you feel that you were not valued as a person. It may also make you feel disempowered and as such may slow down your recovery time.

Activity 1.5 Critical thinking, page 18

Access the Older People's Commissioner for Wales (2010) report, *'Dignified Care': The experiences of older people in hospital in Wales*, to gain a fuller understanding of each of the recommendations. The report can be found at www.olderpeoplewales.com/Libraries/OPCW_Publications/Dignified_Care_Full_Report.sflb.ashx.

You should also be able to get an update on how each local health board in Wales is progressing with regard to implementing the recommendations by accessing the following website: www.olderpeoplewales. com/en/splash.aspx.

Activity 1.6 Critical thinking, page 20

The strategies that could be employed to prevent each type of abuser engaging in abuse in a healthcare setting are as follows.

*   **The reactive abuser** – Ensure staff are regularly supervised, motivated and valued. Particular attention should be paid to staff who appear to be on the edge or 'burnt out'.
*   **The proactive abuser** – This type of abuser is more difficult to deal with. However, vetting procedures may be useful in 'weeding out' those with previous convictions or cautions for abuse. Again, there should be regular supervision and careful monitoring of staff who nurse vulnerable adults, and also a reduction in opportunities for abuse to take place.

Further reading

Deacon, J (1982) *Tongue Tied: Fifty years of friendship in a subnormality hospital.* London: Royal Society for Mentally Handicapped Children and Adults.

This text reports on the life of some people with learning disabilities living in a large learning disability hospital. Some of the language used may be offensive to some but was necessary, as it reflected the language used in the institution at the time.

Froggatt, K, Davies, S and Meyer, J (eds) (2009) *Understanding Care Homes: A research and development perspective.* London: Jessica Kingsley.

This text provides some examples of positive practice in a range of care homes, caring for a variety of vulnerable groups of people.

Pring, J (2011) *Longcare Survivors: The biography of a care scandal.* Layerthorpe: Disability News Service.

This text is useful as it catches up with survivors of abuse to see how they have survived their abusive ordeal.

Useful websites

The following websites are for those organisations that wish to improve the dignity and respect shown to those who are cared for by professionals, particularly in residential or hospital settings.

http://myhomelifemovement.org/about-us

The website of the My Home Life Movement.

www.dignifiedrevolution.org.uk

The website of A Dignified Revolution, ensuring that older people are cared for with dignity and respect.

www.dignityincare.org.uk/DignityCareCampaign

The website of Dignity in Care.

www.midstaffsinquiry.com/assets/docs/Inquiry_Report-Vol1.pdf

www.midstaffsinquiry.com/assets/docs/Inquiry_Report-Vol2.pdf

These are the websites for the two volumes of Mid Staffordshire Inquiry reports discussed in the chapter.

Chapter 2
The meanings of vulnerability

> ### Chapter aims
>
> By the end of this chapter you will be able to:
>
> * discuss the different ways in which 'vulnerable' and 'vulnerability' have been defined;
> * identify the factors that can contribute to vulnerability and also those that can reduce vulnerability;
> * recognise the implications for nursing practice.

Introduction

In health and social care settings the terms 'vulnerable' and 'vulnerability' are commonly used. For example, reference is made to the 'protection of vulnerable adults' and some service users are referred to as being 'vulnerable'. In the context of research mention is often made of 'vulnerable subjects' (see Chapter 10) and, as noted above, the NMC Essential Skills Clusters refer to 'vulnerable situations'. It can therefore be seen that 'vulnerable' is a term that is used to describe someone or something, while vulnerability is the state of being vulnerable. Hoffmaster (2006) highlights how there seems to be an assumption that we all know what vulnerability means, and that we all understand it in the same way. Indeed, it is probably one of those terms that we use every day without really stopping to think what it means. We assume that we understand its meaning(s), and that others hold the same views and perspectives. However, Scanlon and Lee (2007) suggest that there is vagueness and a lack of **consensus** in the literature as to the meaning of vulnerability, implying both a lack of clarity and the presence of differing views and opinions. This chapter will help you to explore some different meanings of vulnerability and encourage you to think about the implications for practice. Before reading further take some time to complete Activity 2.1.

Activity 2.1   *Critical thinking*

Read through the following brief pen pictures of individuals and decide whom you think is vulnerable. Why do you feel they are vulnerable?

Jenny Atkins is 35 years old and works as a freelance illustrator. When she was in her early twenties she was diagnosed as having **bipolar disorder**. Most of the time this is fully controlled by regular medication but sometimes she does experience periods of severe depression, when she finds it difficult to do anything, and also periods of mania, when she rarely sleeps and works non-stop.

George Lewis is 85 years old and lives in a sheltered housing complex where he has his own flat. His mobility is poor as is his eyesight, but generally his health is good. He has all of his shopping delivered, someone comes in to assist him with bathing and someone calls in each day to check that he is OK.

---

continued . . .

James Brookes is 21 years old. Two years ago he had a motorcycle accident, which has left him unable to use his legs. He has an electric wheelchair and an adapted car, and both his home and workplace have been adapted such that he is largely independent. However, as a result of his injuries he does continue to experience some pain that is poorly controlled.

Adele Jones is 19 years old and has **Down's syndrome**. She loves the same things as most 19 year olds and takes great pride in her appearance. She lives at home with her family but has a wide circle of friends and enjoys going out and meeting new people. She has just left school and is in the process of moving to college.

When you have completed this activity turn to the end of the chapter where you will find some suggested areas you may not have considered.

Defining vulnerability

Defining and understanding vulnerability is not just an academic exercise, since if we cannot clearly define a problem then our ability to address it is severely reduced. In particular, if we want to improve practice and develop policies to facilitate this, we need to understand both the nature of the problem and the factors that cause it. Also, we need to acknowledge that, as individuals, we may hold different understandings of vulnerability and what it means to be vulnerable, and this may have particular implications when we as nurses seek to support individuals, families and communities.

Policy definitions

The Department of Health (2010a) suggest that there is no formal definition of vulnerability in healthcare. However, as noted above it is important that understandings of the term are explored in order that appropriate practice is developed. This means that the broader literature needs to be considered.

Within the *No Secrets* policy guidance, which sets out the framework for protecting adults from abuse, a 'vulnerable adult' is defined as being someone:

> *who is or may be in need of community care services by reason of mental or other disability, age or illness; and who is unable to take care of him or herself or is unable to protect him or herself against significant harm or exploitation.*
> (DH, 2000a, pp8–9)

A number of aspects of this definition are worth considering further. It indicates that an individual must either be receiving, or may need to receive, community care services. However, it could be the case that an individual may not receive or require such services but may still be vulnerable. For example, an older person may cope independently but still be vulnerable to financial abuse by family members; or consider the situation of Jenny in Activity 2.1, who may cope without any support from services, but who may nonetheless be vulnerable to abuse and ridicule from other people when she is going through a manic stage of her illness. The definition also suggests that the reason someone may require services is due to the presence of particular personal characteristics/circumstances such as age, disability or illness, which seems to locate the origin of the vulnerability within the person. This use of terminology has been criticised, since people do not like being labelled as being 'vulnerable', and the need for a new statutory definition has been highlighted (Magill et al., 2010). The Department of Health (2000a) definition does go on to identify additional criteria, namely the inability to care for or protect oneself from harm, but even this seems to locate the problem as being an individual deficit. An alternative view might be that someone is vulnerable due to being subjected to significant harm or exploitation by someone, or something. This would lead us to consider what it is that people are vulnerable to.

In fairness, the Department of Health definition is set out for a specific purpose, that is, to identify who is, and who is not, covered by the policies and procedures set up to protect vulnerable adults from abuse (the implications of which are discussed in Chapter 6). As such, it is an official means of setting inclusion and exclusion criteria rather than a broader definition of vulnerability. However, it does highlight some potential difficulties, such as the danger of regarding all members of particular groups as being vulnerable. For example, not all older people are vulnerable, not all disabled people are vulnerable, and there are some people to whom such labels are not applied who are or may be vulnerable. Look back at Activity 2.1: did you consider Adele to be vulnerable just because she has Down's syndrome? Did you consider other aspects of her life and how she might feel about them? As the Department of Health (2011a, p10) highlights, *A person's disability or age does not of itself make the person vulnerable* and Martin (2007) argues that it is something outside the individual that creates vulnerability.

The view expressed by Martin might also be challenged on the grounds that it seems to ignore factors internal to the individual, and if vulnerability is solely created by external factors, a given experience would lead everyone to be vulnerable in the same way, and yet this does not seem to offer sufficient explanation. For example, while everyone admitted to a hospital may, to some degree, be vulnerable, the nature and extent of that vulnerability will differ from one individual to another. Other factors also need to be considered if the complex nature of vulnerability is to be understood.

Vulnerability: a multidimensional concept

Scanlon and Lee (2007) suggest that, in the wider literature, three forms of vulnerability are identified: social, psychological and physical. Table 2.1 sets out some examples of these different forms.

While each of these three areas is presented separately here, they can interact and overlap. For example, illness can be both caused by and made worse by poverty, and our ability to protect ourselves from harm can be affected by our age. Scanlon and Lee (2007), however, do not view vulnerability as a fixed or inevitable state: not all older people are vulnerable and many people with mental health problems cope well on a day-to-day basis. The personal **capacity** of individuals can mediate the effects of vulnerability, which means that increasing personal capacity can be an effective way of reducing vulnerability.

Form of vulnerability	Examples
Social	• Age • Poverty • Cultural issues
Physical	• Physiological imbalances • Impaired resistance to harm • Illness
Psychological	• Low self-esteem • Mental ill health • Fear

Table 2.1 Forms of vulnerability (adapted from Scanlon and Lee, 2007)

The analysis provided by Scanlon and Lee (2007) moves us beyond just looking at individual characteristics such as illness and disability, and introduces additional factors such as social factors and personal resources. For example, two people may have similar levels of depression but one is socially isolated, has limited finances and receives poor support from his general practitioner. In contrast, the other has a small but close circle of friends, good family support and a general practitioner who puts her in touch with a counsellor and an exercise class. The first person is likely to be more vulnerable than the second due to the resources each has access to. Similarly, one person with learning disabilities living in a residential home may be at greater risk of abuse than another, because the latter has relatives who regularly visit and who encourage the person to be assertive, but the former does not have personal visits and after years of living in group settings finds it difficult to speak up.

Vulnerability has many dimensions. Another useful framework is offered by the Department of Health (2011a), which argues that vulnerability is affected by three key factors:

* **personal circumstances** – this will include (but is not limited to) disability or ill health;
* **risks from the environment** – this will include factors such as the level of social contact, a lack of adaptations to meet individual needs and the quality of care received;
* **resilience factors** – this will include support networks, personal strengths and coping mechanisms.

Vulnerability is therefore an interaction between internal and external circumstances and resources that promote resilience. This means that the same circumstances will affect individuals differently and also that identical circumstances may have an impact on an individual in different ways at different times. For example, there are some circumstances that we cope with adequately when we are well but find difficult at times of illness. A person who is visually impaired may cope well within the home as he or she knows where everything is in that environment. However, should the person have to visit a GP surgery, managing the unfamiliar environment could prove difficult and thus the person's vulnerability is increased. Individual vulnerabilities may therefore differ over time (Sellman, 2011) and are also affected by both the physical and psychological environment. Context is therefore an important dimension when considering the appropriateness or otherwise of definitions of vulnerability (Scanlon and Lee, 2007) and, in addition to time and location, culture is an important dimension of context. Different cultures have different beliefs concerning dementia, with some not recognising it as a specific condition but rather as a normal part of the ageing process. In such a situation an older person with dementia may not be seen by his or her family as more vulnerable than other older people. Nurses, however, may find themselves torn between their professional responsibility to promote the safety and well-being of their patients and their desire to respect cultural beliefs. Dilemmas such as this are discussed further in Chapter 3.

Scanlon and Lee (2007) distinguish between actual vulnerability (known factors that cause an individual to be susceptible) and potential vulnerability (circumstances that may cause an individual to be susceptible). This suggests that, if risk factors are known, there is the potential to either eliminate them or to predict and manage them, although Scanlon and Lee do note that, while some factors may be preventable or amenable to adjustment, others (such as social status) may be more complex and difficult to change. De Santis (2008), however, proposes that the concept of vulnerability lacks consistency because it is often used interchangeably with the concept of risk. He maintains that the two concepts are different in that *Vulnerability is the relationship between the person and their environment. Vulnerability is the level at which the culmination of risk factors results in harm for the client* (p282). Thus, one risk factor alone may not have an adverse impact, two may not cause harm, but when others are added an individual becomes vulnerable.

It must also be remembered that the risks associated with vulnerability are not equally distributed throughout society (Delor and Hubert, 2000), hence it is important to remember that some combinations of risks affect some people more than others and also that some people may face greater risks than others. In the situation of a natural disaster such as a flood, where everyone in a given area may be at risk, disabled people may face increased risk due to the difficulties they may face in getting themselves to safety. Flaskerud and Winslow (2010) note how people who have personal resources such as money, power and access to healthcare are able to use these resources to reduce their risk of vulnerability, whereas those who lack such resources are exposed to greater risk and consequently experience poorer health status. The potential for this situation to become a downward spiral is evident, whereby poorer health status exposes people to additional risks, which further diminish their resources and thus increase their vulnerability.

As has been highlighted, vulnerability has been defined in different ways, but for the purpose of this chapter the following definition is offered (see also Figure 2.1):

> *Vulnerability is not an inevitable consequence of particular personal characteristics but rather the complex interaction between the physical and psychological characteristics of an individual and their physical, social, psychological and economic environment. Since it is not inevitable, vulnerability may be reduced and potentially eliminated where it is deemed to be harmful.*

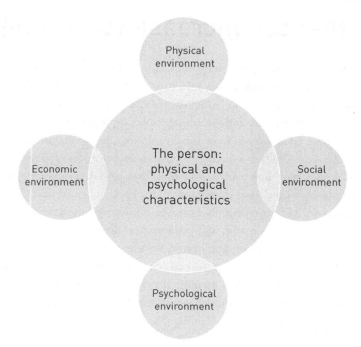

Figure 2.1 A model of vulnerability

Using the framework in Figure 2.1 to assist you, undertake Activity 2.2.

Activity 2.2   *Reflection*

Think about some of the patients and clients with whom you have worked. Can you identify any factors that protected them from or reduced their vulnerability?

Some suggested areas for consideration are given at the end of the chapter.

Activity 2.2 asked you to try to identify some factors that can protect people from vulnerability. This is important within nursing practice as there is a danger that sometimes we focus just on the areas of difficulty or deficit rather than on the strengths that individuals, families and communities possess. By identifying strengths we can support people in recognising their personal strengths and/or in identifying ways they can increase their strengths rather than just applying the label of 'vulnerable adult'. Such an approach is also more likely to have longer-term benefits: as people recognise their personal capacity, their confidence in addressing potential areas of vulnerability increases. It does not deny the existence of vulnerability, but rather encourages an active rather than passive approach.

Factors that can increase vulnerability

It is important that, when seeking to understand vulnerability, we question what it is that an individual, family or community may be vulnerable to. In the context of healthcare, for example, we often talk about individuals or groups being 'vulnerable to' certain illnesses or conditions. Each winter people who are particularly vulnerable to suffering severe effects of the flu virus are encouraged to get vaccinated against it. In healthcare settings, however, one of the factors that can give rise to feelings of vulnerability is a feeling of powerlessness or loss of power. Illness may make some people feel that they have lost control over their lives and that decisions are being taken by other people. It may be that they have to rely on other people more or that they are restricted in terms of what they can do. Most importantly, however, it is important to remember that, no matter how much we aim to work in partnership with patients and their families, there is still a great deal of power attached to professional roles, and even if we aim to work in empowering ways we may still be perceived both by those we support and by others as being more powerful. Simply taking on the role of patient or client may thus increase a person's vulnerability and, in the context of safeguarding, this may make him or her more vulnerable to abuse and neglect.

Take some time to complete Activity 2.3 before reading on.

Activity 2.3 *Critical thinking*

Think about the following settings and consider the factors that may give rise to abuse or neglect:

- an individual's family home;
- a nursing home;
- a hospital ward.

Some outline answers are given at the end of the chapter.

In undertaking Activity 2.3 you will probably have seen that abuse and neglect may occur in a range of settings. Sometimes, however, the factors that cause an individual to be vulnerable can vary and, when considering safeguarding, it is particularly important to identify such factors so that, wherever possible, abuse may be prevented. Particular combinations of factors may lead to individual vulnerability being increased. For example, the Department of Health (2011a) refers to the presence of recurring themes in inquiries concerning failures in care including:

- a lack of patient empowerment particularly in relation to choices concerning their care;
- patients' voices not being heard;
- a lack of preventative and early warning systems, giving rise to abuse and neglect;
- health staff not recognising abuse and neglect;
- safeguarding being viewed as the responsibility of others.

To this list could be added factors such as a lack of staff development, poor recruitment procedures, or isolated staff teams (see also Chapter 1). In developing nursing practice it is therefore important to consider the factors that may give rise to vulnerability, those that may be used to reduce or prevent it, and the significance of time and context. Practice implications will be explored later in this chapter, but first it is important to explore who might (actually or potentially) be vulnerable in healthcare settings.

Who is vulnerable?

The short answer to this question is 'everyone': we all have the potential to be vulnerable whether on a short-term basis or permanently (CARNA, 2005). However, as Sellman (2011) observes, this position does not help us in understanding why particular individuals or groups may require particular consideration in relation to their vulnerability. For this reason he suggests that we should distinguish between ordinary vulnerability (by virtue of being human) and situations where someone is 'more-than-ordinarily' vulnerable. He further adds that, when individuals require the input of health services, they are often 'more-than-ordinarily' vulnerable, hence the importance of nurses being able to recognise and respond appropriately to vulnerability.

As has already been seen, some definitions, such as that offered by the Department of Health (2000a), set clear criteria as to who should be considered vulnerable in specific contexts. In addition, society sometimes assumes that certain groups of people are inevitably vulnerable. For example, some people hold the view that all people with learning disabilities need to be 'looked after' as they are not capable of independent living. Similarly, older people are often thought of as being frail and as having impaired thinking simply by virtue of being a certain age. Clearly, this is not always the case and such views can both stigmatise and, ironically, increase vulnerability through a lack of opportunity to develop or maintain independence. So, while certain people may be at increased risk of vulnerability and harm, labelling entire groups in this manner fails to take account of individual variations and capacities, which (as has already been noted) have an impact upon actual and potential vulnerabilities. Read the case study below and consider whether you feel Mr James is vulnerable and how you have arrived at your assessment of his situation.

Case study: An incorrect assumption of frailty

Albert James is 76 years old and recently he slipped on the ice and fell, breaking his femur. He has been in hospital but is now ready to be discharged. However, as he lives on this own and has no family support close at hand, it has been decided that he should transfer to a local nursing home for a few weeks to enable his physiotherapy to continue and to provide him with additional support. When he arrives at the nursing home he is made welcome, he has a comfortable room and the food is good. From what he can see of the other residents they appear to be very frail and he doesn't really have anyone to interact with except for the staff. While the staff are very pleasant, he does get irritated when they try to do things for him that he is able to do independently. He is also unclear as to why they keep asking when his family will be visiting as they have some things they need to discuss with them. He has asked what these things are, but they say it is nothing for him to worry about. The following weekend, when his son visits, the staff ask him if it is all right for them to wash his father's clothes and to take his photograph for their records. Most worryingly, they ask what should be put on his father's file concerning whether to resuscitate or not should the situation arise.

In the case study above it can be seen that staff had looked at Mr James's age and the fact that he had been admitted to the nursing home and assumed that he was both mentally and physically frail. They had possibly made this assumption based on their knowledge of the clients with whom they usually worked. However, by making this assumption and by seeking to overprotect him, they had increased his vulnerability. In particular, they had made him vulnerable to loss of **autonomy** (see Chapter 3, pages 47–9) and control over his own life. While this case study illustrates how the assumptions of care staff led to them 'taking over' and limiting his control, it is also important to remember that assumptions can lead to healthcare staff overestimating individuals' capacity for self-care and leaving them without assistance. Examples of such 'care' are unfortunately all too common as, for example, we hear of people unable to feed themselves being left to cope alone and their food then being taken away on the assumption that they were not hungry as they hadn't touched it. Such a situation constitutes neglect of the person's nutritional needs and hence is a form of abuse. However, as can be seen, it is not an inevitable consequence of having particular support needs, but rather that an individual is made vulnerable due to an inaccurate assessment of those needs and the failure to provide appropriate support.

The case study also shows how an individual may view themselves as being independent while others view that person as being vulnerable and seek to limit his or her opportunities or to protect him or her. Alternatively, it is possible for an individual to feel very vulnerable, but for others not to recognise this or to ignore it, encouraging him or her instead to take risks. For example, an older person who has had a fall may feel vulnerable and thus is reluctant to mobilise, but the staff view this as important if future vulnerability is to be avoided.

This difference between subjective and objective dimensions of vulnerability can also be seen in relation to situations where there have been allegations of abuse. For example, an adult with learning disabilities who has been giving away most of his or her money to 'friends' may not consider themselves to be vulnerable or abused, yet policy frameworks would identify such behaviour on the part of the 'friends' as financial abuse. Similarly, a young woman with severe depression as a result of experiencing sexual abuse as a child may feel that she has done something wrong to make her abuser act in that way and that she rather than the abuser is to blame.

The interaction between objective and subjective dimensions of vulnerability is complex (Sellman, 2011). Sellman refers to the work of Clarke and Driever (1983), who argue that vulnerability is internal and subjective while risk is external and objective. First, Sellman challenges this position, arguing that with some people (for example, those with a severe learning disability) it may be difficult to determine whether they (subjectively) view themselves as vulnerable, yet most people observing them (objectively) would recognise their vulnerability. Second, he points to the practice of seeking to reduce subjective feelings of vulnerability as an integral part of therapeutic practice. Where the feelings of vulnerability are based on false beliefs, challenging such beliefs may be helpful. For example, where someone with **epilepsy** is reluctant to go out socially, even though he or she has not had a daytime seizure for many years, it may be appropriate to challenge the person's perceptions about his or her vulnerability in social situations, and to encourage the person to try going out more.

However, where the feelings of vulnerability are an accurate reflection of reality, seeking to reduce them may give rise to feelings of invulnerability and invincibility, which themselves can lead to unwise risk taking and increased vulnerability. For example, if a young person suffers extreme anxiety in social situations, fearing everyone wants to harm him or her, it might be helpful to work with that person to alter his or her beliefs and increase his or her self-confidence. However, if the person is led to develop the belief that he or she will not be harmed in any social situation, the person may place themselves in situations of unwise risk. Similarly, if there is a strong possibility of the young person being confronted with harmful situations, it would not be appropriate to encourage him or her to increase social activity without also enabling the person to develop personal safety measures or different social activities.

Of course, the situation can become even more complex when, for example, a young woman with learning disabilities wishes to go out with her sister and friends to a night club and does not understand why she may be more vulnerable in such an environment. Her parents refuse to let her go, to which she responds by becoming very angry, accusing them of treating her like a child. Why is her sister allowed to go and yet they stop her? While the individual's desire to take part in social activities can be understood (and many parents would worry at their teenagers going to clubs), increased parental concerns about personal safety can also be understood. Our own assessment of our vulnerability and the assessment of others may be very different. Similarly, professional assessments of vulnerability may be very different from the views of the individuals with whom such professionals work. Take some time to work through Activity 2.4.

Activity 2.4   *Critical thinking*

- Think about the nature of vulnerability and try to list as many factors as you can that may make people feel vulnerable.
- Try also to think about situations in which you feel vulnerable. What is it that makes you feel this way?

There are some comments regarding this activity at the end of the chapter.

Recognising our own vulnerability

If everyone is vulnerable, it follows that we as nurses are also vulnerable. This is true in our everyday lives, but particularly so in relation to our professional lives. In Activity 2.4 some of the situations you identified in which you feel vulnerable may have related to your personal life while others relate to your work. For example, in our work we bear witness to some very difficult and harrowing situations: we can be subjected to physical or verbal abuse, we may undertake physically demanding work that places us at risk of injury and we may be bullied by colleagues. Often, however, as nurses we are expected not to show our vulnerability, which can mean that we do not recognise our own vulnerability. Activity 2.5 asks you to think about this issue and how it might be addressed.

Activity 2.5   *Critical thinking*

Think of the settings in which nurses work and the types of work they undertake.

- Which factors might increase their vulnerability?
- How might their vulnerability be reduced?

Some outline answers are given at the end of the chapter.

In Activity 2.5 you may have managed to identify both factors that give rise to vulnerability and some actions that could be taken to reduce such vulnerability. You may also have been able to think about some of the situations in which you have found yourself and perhaps how you might handle such situations differently in the future. Malone (2000) argues that, while choosing to be a nurse can be a way of increasing control over the uncertainties of life, it also brings people face to face with their fears concerning these uncertainties. Despite the fact that nurses might be viewed as being at greater risk of harm than other occupational groups, Sellman (2011) argues that they are not 'more-than-ordinarily' vulnerable, as usually they have the capacity for self-protection. He argues that they are at risk of exposure to occupational hazards and that they are witness to the 'more-than-ordinary' vulnerability of others on a regular basis within their work. It may be possible to reduce or remove any occupational hazards. Witnessing the vulnerability of other people, however, is a common feature of nursing that highlights the importance of us developing effective coping mechanisms. If you are a student nurse this may be a particular challenge, as you may not have had much experience of such situations or opportunities to develop your coping mechanisms. You may, therefore, feel particularly vulnerable but feel that you should be able to cope. Being willing to recognise our own vulnerability rather than being ashamed of it is, however, an important first step in being able to develop appropriate coping strategies. As Hoffmaster (2006) argues, *none of us is invincible.*

Case study: Recognising our own vulnerability

Luke Samuels is a second-year student nurse. He is 34 years old, is married and has two young children. Just before his placement with the district nursing team his father died from pancreatic cancer and, although Luke had been with him when he died, the time between diagnosis and death had been quick and so the family had not had long to adjust to what was happening. When he started the placement he didn't want to appear difficult or weak and so didn't mention his recent bereavement to his mentor. However, one of the patients they visited was a young man of a similar age to him who also had two young children and who had returned home from hospital as he wished to die at home. Luke finds this situation very difficult and tries to cope, but this results in him becoming quite withdrawn and uncommunicative. Noticing this, his mentor challenges him, and asks if there is anything wrong. Initially he says that everything is fine, but then breaks down and talks about his experience and his feelings. They discuss this and make arrangements for him to receive some additional support. As a result, Luke feels better able to work with the patient and takes pride in trying to make his final days as comfortable as possible.

Working to support people who are vulnerable can be very stressful and over time this can lead to burnout. However, as Sellman (2011) observes, there does not seem to be any evidence that nurses working within **palliative care** settings have higher levels of burnout than those working elsewhere, and yet the very nature of their work means that they work on a daily basis with people who are at the end of their lives. Some emergency nurses in Malone's (2000) study used strategies such as distancing themselves from situations as a means of coping, whereas others actively engaged with their patients and their suffering. While distancing may afford a degree of protection to nurses it can, unfortunately, also lead to dehumanisation of patients and neglect of their care. Malone thus refers to the 'paradox' of vulnerability whereby *it can be either bond or barrier between nurse and patient* (p9). Effective coping thus requires that nurses recognise their own vulnerability and Hoffmaster (2006) argues that to be able to truly care for others requires that we recognise our common humanity and common vulnerability. Vulnerability in this context thus becomes a strength rather than a sign of weakness since it allows us to develop **empathy** and understanding. Supportive strategies such as debriefing after particularly stressful clinical events, clinical supervision, use of a personal tutorial system and the use of support services such as counselling can all be useful ways of recognising our vulnerability and addressing it in a constructive way.

> **Research summary: Meanings of vulnerability**
>
> Stenbock-Hunt and Sarvimaki (2011) report a study of 16 nurses in Finland who were experienced in working with older people. The study sought to explore participants' meanings of vulnerability. Interviews were recorded, transcribed and then analysed using a **qualitative** interpretative approach. One core theme (vulnerability as being human and having feelings) and six sub-themes (having feelings, experiencing moral indignation, being harmed, having courage, protecting oneself, and maturing and developing) emerged. Vulnerability was viewed not only as a burden being associated with negative feelings, but also as a resource both for improving care and for personal development. While the limitations of the study are noted, it concluded that *Only if nurses are able to deal with their own vulnerability will they be able to develop an existential and ethical attitude and encounter older persons' vulnerability* (p40).

Implications for practice

If we accept that everyone is vulnerable, it follows that in considering the implications for practice we have to determine the implications for the individuals, families and communities with whom we work, and whom we seek to support. However, we also need to consider the implications for how we support colleagues, and seek and accept support for ourselves: if we as nurses are vulnerable ourselves, this will affect (either positively or negatively) the care and support we are able to provide to others. Take some time to work through Activity 2.6.

| Activity 2.6 | *Decision making and communication* |

- How would you assess someone's vulnerability?
- What factors would you consider and which sources of information would you use?

Some outline answers are given at the end of the chapter.

In practice we need to be able to *recognise* factors that may increase vulnerability. Think back to Figure 2.1 and consider how personal characteristics (both physical and psychological) might interact with social, physical, economic and psychological environments to give rise to vulnerability. Indeed, such a framework might usefully form the basis of an assessment. Having identified such factors we also need to recognise their significance within the particular context in which we are working. For example, we need to understand that over-reliance on complex written information may make people with learning disabilities more vulnerable or that loud, busy environments may increase the agitation and confusion of people with dementia. We need to understand that a person who has recently suffered a traumatic event may be vulnerable to adverse psychological consequences even if they are not apparent at present. We also need to understand that our perception of vulnerability may differ from that of others and that an apparently similar combination of circumstances may affect people very differently.

Accurate, comprehensive and timely assessment is therefore required in order that actual vulnerability can be identified and situations of potential vulnerability are, wherever possible, predicted and averted. In relation to looking after ourselves and supporting our colleagues we need to recognise factors that may make us feel vulnerable, and where the circumstances cannot be altered or avoided (for example, being confronted by people in distress) we need to identify commonly occurring situations and work proactively with others to develop our coping mechanisms.

We need to be able to *respond* appropriately when we encounter people in vulnerable situations or who feel themselves to be vulnerable. For example, continuing the examples previously discussed, we need to make sure that we have easy-to-read information available for people with learning disabilities when they attend health clinics, we need to make sure that there are quiet waiting areas for people with dementia when they attend Accident and Emergency (A&E) departments and we need to make sure that people suffering the effects of trauma are provided with appropriate specialist help. We also need to be able to respond at an emotional level, recognising others' distress and responding in a valuing and supportive manner and offering opportunities for individuals to talk about and explore their feelings.

We also need to be able to regularly *review* situations to determine levels of vulnerability in dynamic and changing situations. For example, someone who has a terminal illness may be vulnerable to infection at one stage due to the effects of **chemotherapy**, at another time may be vulnerable to depression as he or she tries to adjust to the situation, and at another time may be vulnerable to extreme levels of pain. This means that the person's situation needs constantly reassessing, as what reduces vulnerability at one stage may not be effective at another.

This book is about safeguarding and so the importance of recognising, responding and reviewing needs to be carefully considered in this context. The issues will be expanded upon elsewhere in the book, but here it is relevant to note the importance of being alert to signs of abuse and neglect, being aware of the appropriate responses and being alert to the need to review both situations and actions taken on a regular basis (see Figure 2.2).

It is also important to consider whether a certain degree of vulnerability can be helpful in some situations (for example, it is suggested in the previous section that recognising our own vulnerability can be important in the development of an empathetic and caring attitude). This needs to be countered by recognising that feelings of invincibility can also be problematic since they may lead individuals to take unwarranted and unnecessary risks. Clearly, however, most people would want to avoid situations in which they are 'more-than-ordinarily' vulnerable. Where factors that may give rise to vulnerability can be predicted, it may therefore be important to work with clients in order to increase their resilience. This could, for example, include actions such as ensuring that they have appropriately trained support at key times, providing them with communication aids so that they can make their views known to others or reducing their anxiety levels through desensitisation programmes. Increasing resilience to abuse is particularly important and could include strategies such as assertiveness training, provision of information concerning rights or increasing awareness of what constitutes abuse. It may also include working to strengthen people's support networks.

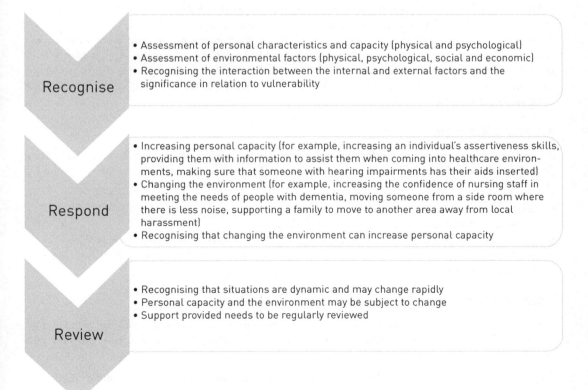

Recognise
- Assessment of personal characteristics and capacity (physical and psychological)
- Assessment of environmental factors (physical, psychological, social and economic)
- Recognising the interaction between the internal and external factors and the significance in relation to vulnerability

Respond
- Increasing personal capacity (for example, increasing an individual's assertiveness skills, providing them with information to assist them when coming into healthcare environments, making sure that someone with hearing impairments has their aids inserted)
- Changing the environment (for example, increasing the confidence of nursing staff in meeting the needs of people with dementia, moving someone from a side room where there is less noise, supporting a family to move to another area away from local harassment)
- Recognising that changing the environment can increase personal capacity

Review
- Recognising that situations are dynamic and may change rapidly
- Personal capacity and the environment may be subject to change
- Support provided needs to be regularly reviewed

Figure 2.2 Addressing vulnerability in practice

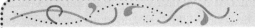

Chapter summary

This chapter has explored a number of different definitions of vulnerability and has challenged the assumption that we all understand vulnerability in the same way. It has been argued that vulnerability is a complex concept, that everyone is vulnerable, and that vulnerability is influenced by the interaction of internal and external factors. Since vulnerability may be reduced or eliminated, nurses, who work regularly with people who are particularly vulnerable, have a key role to play in recognising, responding to and reviewing vulnerability. Also, since nurses themselves may be vulnerable, they have a responsibility to recognise and respond to their own vulnerability and that of their colleagues.

Activities: Brief outline answers

Activity 2.1 Critical thinking, pages 26–7

In undertaking this activity you may have looked at the brief outlines provided and concluded that all of the individuals are vulnerable by virtue of their age, disability or health needs. However, a closer look reveals that, while the individuals concerned may be potentially vulnerable, a number of measures are in place to reduce their vulnerability, such as the provision of personal support, services, aids and adaptations. It might also be important to consider whether, if asked, the individuals concerned feel vulnerable. Nonetheless, it is important to note that there is the potential for vulnerability. For example, what if Jenny experiences a period of severe depression, feels unable to go out and has no friends or family to support her? What if James has to go into hospital for assessment of his pain and is told that he cannot take his electric wheelchair with him? He would then be dependent upon staff to meet his needs and his vulnerability may increase. Vulnerability is therefore a complex issue.

Activity 2.2 Reflection, page 31

A number of factors may protect individuals from vulnerability or reduce the impact of vulnerability. Some you may have identified include:

- good support networks of family and/or friends;
- financial resources;
- well-planned packages of care that meet individual needs;
- personal coping mechanisms such as assertiveness, good self-esteem and self-awareness;
- legal provisions such as the Mental Health Act 1983 and the Mental Capacity Act 2005 (see Chapter 6 for further details).

Activity 2.3 Critical thinking, page 32

Some factors that may lead to abuse and neglect may be common to all settings, while others may differ between informal (home) and formal (nursing home and hospital) care. Some factors you may have identified include:

- differences in power whereby the abuser is in a powerful position relative to the person for whom he or she is caring;
- carers lacking the appropriate value base and/or the necessary skills;
- carers and those for whom they care lacking awareness as to what constitutes abuse and neglect;

- a lack of monitoring;
- stress;
- people who require support lacking a voice or, even if they do speak up, not being believed;
- low self-esteem and self-worth.

Activity 2.4 Critical thinking, page 35

To some extent what makes us feel vulnerable will inevitably be individual. However, there are some situations and experiences that commonly give rise to feelings of vulnerability. These include:

- having an illness that interferes with our usual day-to-day functioning;
- being admitted to hospital – even the process of changing into nightclothes and going to bed may make us feel more vulnerable;
- being in a situation where nothing is being explained to us even though we know it affects us;
- loss and bereavement;
- being in new situations;
- feeling that we lack the knowledge and skills needed for a situation.

Activity 2.5 Critical thinking, page 36

In thinking about the ways in which nurses might be vulnerable, some of the things you may have considered might include:

- not feeling adequately prepared for a situation;
- dealing with patients and relatives who become verbally or physically abusive;
- levels of responsibility and/or dealing with very complex situations;
- low staffing levels;
- lone working in a community setting;
- witnessing the vulnerability of other people and sometimes not being able to do anything to reduce it;
- having to cope with difficulties and challenges in our own lives while supporting others going through difficult situations that may sometimes be similar to our own circumstances.

Activity 2.6 Decision making and communication, page 38

In assessing people's vulnerability you could use the framework offered by the Department of Health (2011a) as discussed earlier in the chapter. You would therefore try to determine the following.

- What are their personal circumstances? This could include consideration of factors such as the presence of any disability, illness and/or personal support needs. It might also include factors such as their normal living circumstances and their personal views, beliefs and wishes.
- What risks can be determined in their environment? This might include aspects such as the frequency and nature of social contacts (not all may be positive and some may be abusive), physical barriers within the environment that have a negative impact on mobility and self-care, and environments that may have a negative impact on the psychological vulnerability of an individual.
- What factors are present that may reduce vulnerability? This may include aspects such as personal strengths, social networks and financial resources.
- In seeking to gather this information it would be important to speak with the individual concerned, any relevant family or carers and other professionals who regularly support that person. In addition, it would be important to use good observational skills. Any differences in perception should be noted.

Further reading

Abley, C, Bond, J and Robinson, L (2011) Improving inter-professional practice for vulnerable older people: gaining a better understanding of vulnerability, *Journal of Inter-professional Care*, 25(5): 359–65.

Fyffe, DC, Botticello, AL and Myaskovsky, L (2011) Vulnerable groups living with spinal cord injury, *Topics in Spinal Cord Injury Rehabilitation*, 17(2): 1–9.

Parley, F (2011) What does vulnerability mean? *British Journal of Learning Disabilities*, 39(4): 266–76.

Useful websites

http://patients-association.com

The Patients Association campaigns for improvements in patient care and has published a number of reports highlighting the vulnerability of patients.

www.mencap.org.uk

Mencap campaigns for better support for people with learning disabilities and for recognition of their rights. A key area of campaigning has focused on highlighting their vulnerability to poor healthcare provision.

Chapter 3
Ethical frameworks and principles

NMC Standards for Pre-registration Nursing Education

This chapter will address the following competencies:

Domain 1: Professional values

1. All nurses must practice with confidence according to *The Code: Standards of conduct, performance and ethics for nurses and midwives* (NMC, 2008a), and within other recognised ethical and legal frameworks. They must be able to recognise and address ethical challenges relating to people's choices and decision making about their care, and act within the law to help them and their families and carers find acceptable solutions.

Domain 2: Communication and interpersonal skills

8. All nurses must respect individual rights to confidentiality and keep information secure and confidential in accordance with the law and relevant ethical and regulatory frameworks taking account of local protocols. They must also actively share personal information with others when the interests of safety and protection override the need for confidentiality.

NMC Essential Skills Clusters

This chapter will address the following ESCs:

Cluster: Care, compassion and communication

2. People can trust the newly registered graduate nurse to engage in person centred care empowering people to make choices about how their needs are met when they are unable to meet them for themselves.

3. People can trust the newly registered graduate nurse to respect them as individuals and strive to help them preserve their dignity at all times.

4. People can trust a newly registered graduate nurse to engage with them and their family or carers within their cultural environments in an acceptant and anti-discriminatory manner free from harassment and exploitation.

7. People can trust the newly registered graduate nurse to protect and keep as confidential all information relating to them.

8. People can trust the newly registered graduate nurse to gain their consent based on sound understanding and informed choice prior to any intervention and that their rights in decision making and consent will be respected and upheld.

> ## Chapter aims
>
> By the end of this chapter you will be able to:
>
> * review different ethical perspectives and principles;
> * recognise their relevance to safeguarding in practice;
> * understand how ethical dilemmas can arise;
> * utilise an ethical framework to assist decision making in practice.

Introduction

This chapter will introduce you to some key aspects of ethics and ethical practice. It is beyond the scope of this book to provide a comprehensive overview of ethics, and you are referred to other sources for such information (see further reading at the end of this chapter). Nonetheless, as Weaver et al. (2008) argue, it is important for nurses to develop 'ethical sensitivity' if they are to be able to respond in a moral manner to the vulnerability of patients and clients. This suggests that, if we are to safeguard people from abuse and neglect, we must have an understanding of key ethical perspectives and principles, so that we can recognise when such principles are at risk of being ignored, and so that ethical principles can inform our decision making.

> ## Activity 3.1   *Reflection*
>
> Before reading the rest of this chapter, take a few minutes to reflect on why you decided to become a nurse.
>
> * What did you hope to achieve?
> * What did you feel you could bring to the role?
> * Do you feel your values have changed at all as a result of your nursing experience?
>
> *Keep your answers in mind as you read through the chapter and then take a look at the outline answers at the end of the chapter.*

What do we mean by 'ethics'?

Ethics is a subject of philosophical study and debate. It can also be a framework within which we live our everyday lives, including our professional lives. In this sense it can be seen very much as an 'applied' subject. Thompson et al. (2006) define applied ethics in the context of nursing as acting responsibly, appropriately and effectively, while being able to provide a clear rationale for decisions and actions by reference to standards that are commonly accepted.

There are a few important aspects of this definition to consider. First, it suggests that we need to act 'responsibly, appropriately and effectively' but this, in turn, means that we need some standards against which our behaviour can be judged. Indeed, the definition goes on to refer to 'commonly accepted' standards, which might include frameworks such as the law and our professional code of conduct (NMC, 2008a). However, elsewhere Seedhouse (2009) argues that ethics does not provide us with just one view of what is right and what is wrong. This suggests that, while there are some areas where most people would agree as to what is considered right and wrong, acceptable or unacceptable, there may also be some different views. Why this should be the case is explained by Barker (2012), who identifies that most definitions of ethics include reference to the system of moral values, which explains why we believe that something is the right thing to do. Awareness of our moral values enables us to provide the justification for our actions (Thompson et al., 2006), which is an essential part of ethical nursing practice; we must not only be able to act in an ethical manner, but we must be able to provide a rationale for our decisions and our behaviour.

Fry and Johnstone (2008) suggest that values are standards that are considered important and desirable. They are expressed through behaviours that individuals seek to maintain or support and each individual has a system in which his or her values are organised into a hierarchical order of importance to that person.

A value is therefore something that we, as individuals, feel is important and that guides us to behave in particular ways. Examples might include valuing honesty, respecting other cultures and supporting freedom of speech. However, as Fry and Johnstone (2008) suggest, some values are more important to us than others, they may change over time, and there may be clashes in particular situations. Imagine a situation in which one patient is making culturally offensive comments about another – would the value of respecting other cultures or that of freedom of speech be more important to you in deciding how to respond?

Fry and Johnstone (2008) also suggest that values can be recognised at a variety of levels, including personal, professional and cultural levels. Tensions can arise for individuals when clashes occur between values existing at these different levels. Nurses may enter the profession because they feel that the professional values of nursing reflect their personal values of respecting individuals and compassion. As their careers progress they find that, while this is generally the case, there are some aspects of the nursing role that create conflict with their cultural values. For example, it could be that in one nurse's culture it is customary for the extended family to be present when an individual dies and to stay with him or her during the final hours offering prayers. However, when someone dies within an open ward environment it is difficult to respect requests for this to happen due to issues such as space, and the need to provide a quiet environment for other patients. In this situation the nurse may experience distress as she feels unable to provide care that respects her cultural values and those of some patients.

Specific values may also be evident at the level of the organisation. In some instances these may be explicit, but in other situations they may be evident as part of the culture rather than written into any policy document. Policy documents may therefore set out mission statements and goals that stress the importance of high-quality, person-centred care delivered at the times when patients need it. However, the limited funds available to provide such care may result in a situation whereby the need to contain costs takes precedence over the desire to provide timely care. This situation can lead to great stress for nurses who feel themselves unable to deliver the care they wish – professional care that reflects their personal values. Indeed, in one study nurses reported that staffing patterns that had a negative impact upon their work was the most stressful ethical and patient care issue they encountered (Ulrich et al., 2010). This stress arose because the nurses in the study felt that low staffing levels meant that they could not provide ethical patient care.

Ethical perspectives and principles

A review of any textbook concerning ethics will show that many ethical theories and perspectives have been proposed. They provide us with different ways of analysing and understanding situations, and act as a guide to decision making and action. As noted earlier in the chapter, it is not possible here to discuss these in detail, but an overview is provided to help you understand how consideration of these different positions can assist you in practice.

Thompson et al. (2006) classify the ethical theories into three main groups: those that are concerned with 'causes', those that are concerned with 'means' and those that are concerned with 'ends'. If the focus of an ethical theory is on 'causes' it will be concerned with those things that cause us to act in a particular way. Another way of putting this would be to say that such theories would be concerned with what motivates us to act in a specific manner, in a particular situation. Here, the relevance of values (as discussed earlier in the chapter) can be seen, since we may be motivated to act as a result of our personal, cultural or professional values. Of course, our motivation may also result from a combination of these values.

Case study: Conflicting values

Consider the situation in which you are supporting Angela Francis, a young woman who is physically disabled, and her partner, who wish to become parents. Their family and some health professionals have made it plain that they do not feel this is a good idea. The reasons they give include things such as not believing that Angela will be able to cope, that it will not be good for her health, and that the child will be at risk. You might reflect on why you feel so strongly that you should support the couple, and your reasons might include the fact that you are motivated by the belief that people have a right to be parents, and that the decisions of the couple should be respected.

Those theories that are concerned with the 'means' focus on how we act. In a practice setting this might include aspects such as whether care is provided in a respectful manner or whether measures are taken to try to promote/maintain independence. It might also support us in considering whether certain approaches/interventions can be ethically justified. When looking at how people act it is interesting to note, however, that their actions may not always match what they state to be their values. For example, in a study undertaken in a Norwegian nursing home, observation revealed that, while values such as respect and **self-determination** were well known and accepted by staff, they were not always evident within the care observed (Solum et al., 2008).

In everyday language we use the phrase 'the end justifies the means' and this highlights how important it is for us not only to consider how we do things but also to be clear as to what it is that we want to achieve. Indeed, our choice of actions may be decided by what we feel will be the outcomes and what our goals are. The group of ethical theories that focuses on the 'ends' thus encourages us to look at what our goals are, and what the consequences of our actions are likely to be. It is also important to consider what the outcomes of not taking action are likely to be, since inaction as well as action has consequences. Take some time to work through Activity 3.2.

Activity 3.2   *Critical thinking*

Think of a practice situation you have recently encountered and critically analyse it by considering the following.

- What motivated you and others to act in a particular way?
- What influenced how you behaved in the situation?
- What happened as a result of your actions and those of others?
- Were the consequences considered before deciding on a course of action?

Some outline answers are given at the end of the chapter.

In completing Activity 3.2 you may have thought not only about your values and those of others, but also about other principles that guide your behaviour. Some values and principles that may be relevant in clinical situations are highlighted at the end of the chapter. Wheeler (2012) argues that nurses require *certain ethical and morally acceptable guiding principles* (p179) to underpin their practice. He further argues that codes of professional conduct provide one source of information to assist them in identifying such principles. Nonetheless, a broader understanding is also required, and one commonly used framework of ethical principles is that offered by Beauchamp and Childress (2009). They identify four key principles, namely **autonomy**, **non-maleficence**, **beneficence** and **justice**. You may not be familiar with these words as they are not commonly used in everyday language. An explanation of their meanings will, however, show you that they are principles with which you should be familiar (they are also included in the glossary).

Autonomy

Autonomy is concerned with respecting the right of individuals to be self-determining: it is customary within modern society to respect the right of adults to make decisions concerning their own lives. Indeed, it is a right that is highly valued in many societies and it is linked to other highly valued attributes such as independence. It is seen as a core feature of being human, and a lack of autonomy is often viewed negatively and, in some instances, leads to people being somehow less than human. This has significant implications in relation to safeguarding, as examples are seen of dehumanising care being provided, particularly to people whose autonomy may be impaired. A lack of autonomy also makes people relatively powerless, which places them at risk of abuse and neglect. In the context of healthcare, autonomy has particular significance, as it relates to issues such as **consent** and **confidentiality**.

If we are to support patients and clients to exercise autonomy we need to recognise that there are a number of factors that can influence their capacity to act autonomously. First, in order for them to make decisions in an informed manner, we need to ensure that the people we support have access to accurate, balanced and timely information in a format they can understand. Second, we need to recognise that there is a range of factors that may limit the extent to which their expressed views and opinions are respected by other people, such as their families and other members of the healthcare team. For example, others may dismiss their views on the basis of age, gender, culture and religion – for example, 'they are too young to know what's good for them'. In such circumstances we as nurses can have an important role to play as advocates: listening to the views and wishes of patients and making sure that they are heard by others. The final area we need to consider in relation to autonomy is that there are situations when an individual's capacity to act autonomously is impaired either on a temporary basis (such as when someone is sedated post-operatively or is in an acute phase of psychosis), or on a longer-term basis (such as when someone has a severe learning disability or has advanced dementia). In such circumstances it is important that appropriate legal measures are taken (see Chapter 6). However, it is also important to consider the ethical implications if we seek to act in someone's **best interests**. Work through Activity 3.3 before reading on.

Activity 3.3 — *Decision making and communication*

Imagine you are a student nurse working on an acute mental health unit. You have been working on the unit for a few weeks now and you have developed a good relationship with a patient, Sally Thomas, who was admitted with severe depression. At first, Sally was very withdrawn, and said very little to anyone. Over time her mood has lifted, and though she still doesn't interact a great deal with others, she does speak with you. She has talked about her family and about her worries for them. She has also said in the past that she feels she has let them down, and that they would be better off without her. This information has been passed back to the qualified staff on the unit. Today, however, you spend some time talking with her and in the course of conversation she says that she has decided that she needs to kill herself. As soon as she says this she states that you must not tell anyone, adding that she knows you will keep her secret safe as you respect her right to make her own decisions.

- How will you respond to Sally's disclosure and her request?
- How will you justify your actions?

Some key points are included at the end of the chapter to assist you in completing this activity.

In Activity 3.3 you will probably have decided that, while you do generally respect Sally's views, in this instance you need to act in her best interests, and to tell senior staff what she has said. When we act on behalf of others in their best interests (but not at their request) to try to protect them from harm or to benefit them, we may be said to be acting paternalistically (from **paternalism**) (Edwards, 2009). If those other people have the capacity to make their own decisions, they may feel aggrieved that someone else is making decisions about their lives. Think, for example, of times when other people have acted on your behalf, believing that they were acting in your best interests. How did you feel? Did you agree with the decisions they made? If the other person does not have capacity, or appears not to have capacity, there may be a temptation automatically to make decisions on his or her behalf. This may be ethically justified in order to prevent harm (although it needs to be remembered that all of us at some time have made unwise decisions). Alternatively, it may be that assumptions have inappropriately been made about the individual's capacity on the basis, for example, of age or appearance, such that others are making decisions about the person's life when he or she could (with appropriate support) be able to make at least some decisions independently. When acting in someone's best interests it is therefore important that we are able to justify why we have acted paternalistically (Edwards, 2009).

Read through the case study below and then complete Activity 3.4. This will help you to consider how our practice can assist in promoting greater autonomy for the people we support, and the importance of avoiding assumptions.

Case study: A loss of autonomy

Eric Holmes is 85 years old. He suffers from chronic respiratory problems and has recently had a stroke. This has left him with limited mobility and with little speech. He has recently moved into a nursing home because of his increased support needs but he is having difficulty settling in. The nursing staff have observed that he seems to be getting very agitated and, particularly at mealtimes, he becomes rather aggressive, spitting his food at staff. They assume that this is all part of his current health state and so try to manage it rather than trying to understand it.

Unfortunately, when he came to the home very little information came with him from the hospital. He doesn't have any family living close by but a friend who used to live nearby does visit regularly. He is very concerned about Eric as he used to be such an independent man with very clear ideas about what he wanted and didn't want.

Activity 3.4   *Decision making and communication*

Read through the case study above. Imagine you are a nurse working in this home who is concerned about Mr Holmes. How might you try to increase his autonomy?

You can compare the suggestions you make with those included at the end of the chapter.

Non-maleficence

Non-maleficence is concerned with seeking to ensure that harm does not occur to patients and clients. You might feel that this should be such an obvious part of healthcare practice that it does not need mentioning. Experience shows us, however, that unfortunately harm does occur on a regular basis within the healthcare system. Such harm may be physical and/or psychological. The occurrences of such events due to malicious and deliberate actions on the part of individuals are, thankfully, rare. When they do occur they are usually high profile and are much discussed in the media. Examples include cases such as that of nurse Beverley Allitt (mentioned in Chapter 1), who harmed children within her care, and that of Dr Harold Shipman, a GP who killed a number of his older patients. At the time of writing, 11 members of staff have pleaded guilty to the abuse of people with learning disabilities at Winterbourne View, a privately run hospital unit for people with learning disabilities and challenging behaviour (see Chapter 1, pages 12–13).

Recently, other examples of alleged harm within healthcare settings have also come to public attention. The Patients Association has published a series of reports that focus on patient stories (for example, Patients Association, 2011). While some positive aspects of care are noted, failings in care leading to harm to patients are also evident. Similarly, Mencap (2012) has highlighted a number of instances where it is suggested that failures in care have led both to harm and to the deaths of people with learning disabilities. Reading reports such as these highlights how, while individual acts may not have a significant impact on their own, they can very easily contribute to greater harm as the action or inaction of one practitioner compounds those of other people. Unfortunately, it would seem that, while practitioners may not set out to cause harm to their patients and clients, such harm can and does occur within the healthcare system. This reinforces the importance of all nurses remaining alert to the potential for harm, and being able to take action to avert or limit such harm.

Beneficence

At the beginning of this chapter we asked you to think about why you decided to become a nurse. It is possible that one of the reasons you identified was that you wanted to help other people and to 'do good'. This is the basis of beneficence, which is concerned with seeking to ensure that our patients and clients gain the maximum benefit from the nursing care we provide, and from wider packages of care provision. In determining what might be seen as 'maximum benefit', nurses need to take account of a range of factors such as the best available evidence (see Chapter 10), the availability of resources, the demands upon these resources and, most importantly, the views and preferences of individual patients and clients. For example, a multidisciplinary team may feel that a series of counselling sessions would benefit an individual who is recovering from severe depression, but the individual concerned does not hold the same view. In such a situation it is possible that counselling may not achieve the maximum benefit if it is provided. This example also demonstrates how there can be tension between one ethical principle and another: should the principle of beneficence be given more weight than the principle of autonomy (respecting the wishes of the patient)?

Wheeler (2012) also notes how the different ethical principles relate to one another by arguing that, in deciding what will achieve most benefit for an individual, the nurse needs to consider the balance between risks and benefits. Here it can be seen that both non-maleficence and beneficence need to be considered: potential benefits should outweigh the potential risks. Consider an older person who wishes to be discharged from hospital. He or she is medically fit to be discharged and it is felt that going home will not only benefit the person psychologically, but will also reduce the potential risk of harm such as hospital-acquired infections. However, since being ill the person has lost the ability to perform certain aspects of self-care. In particular, there is some loss of mobility, and he or she would find it difficult to attend to hygiene and nutritional needs. In such a situation it would be important to ensure that adaptations are made to the home as required and that an appropriate package of care is put in place before discharge. Safeguarding would be achieved by consideration of both the risks and benefits.

Justice

Justice is the fourth ethical principle identified by Beauchamp and Childress (2009). Many people think of justice narrowly as relating to the law, but while the law has an important role to play, in this context justice has a wider meaning. In an ethical sense justice relates to issues of fairness, equality and equity and it requires that we value difference and diversity (Wheeler, 2012). It is therefore concerned with who gets what resources, how we make such judgements, and what the effects are of such decisions. In nursing practice this could relate to such concerns as how we allocate staff so that patients receive support that is appropriate to their individual needs. If we accept that individuals have different needs, this means that, if we just allocate the same level of support to all patients, we will not be acting in a fair manner. Consider the situation described in the following case study concerning Princy Joseph.

In practice, you may also have come across colleagues who believe some patients to be less deserving of support than others and this is reflected in their behaviour towards them. In such instances their behaviour might be questioned on ethical grounds: are they ensuring that justice is upheld?

Case study: Should everyone be treated the same?

Princy Joseph is 24 years old. She enjoys listening to music and going out in the car. She does not communicate verbally but her family understands how she makes her needs known. She has severe learning disabilities and complex health needs. She has regular epileptic seizures and recurrent respiratory infections, and she has to be carefully positioned so as to reduce problems with her breathing and to prevent deformities of her limbs. She has recently been admitted to a new hospital as she has another respiratory infection. On admission the nurse in charge of the ward tells her parents not to worry as the staff do not discriminate against disabled people on the ward: they treat everybody the same. Her parents are very concerned.

Activity 3.5   *Critical thinking*

Using the four ethical principles proposed by Beauchamp and Childress (2009), analyse the above case study.

- Why do you think Princy's parents are concerned?
- Is the ward correct to 'treat everybody the same'?
- Do you feel that Princy could be at risk?

Some outline answers are given at the end of the chapter.

Duties and rights

Other principles that are important within the context of nursing are those that relate to duties and rights. As Thompson et al. (2006) point out, there has long been an emphasis within nursing on a '**duty of care**', but discussion of patients' rights is a more recent development. Some rights are established within legislation and these will be discussed in Chapter 6. The principles of rights and duty are related in that, if one party has a right or claim to something, another party has a duty or responsibility to address that claim. Within nursing, for example, patients have a right to be treated in a manner that respects their dignity and that safeguards them from harm. This means nurses have a duty to provide dignified and respectful care while making every effort to protect patients from harm. While, at one level, this appears relatively straightforward, closer examination reveals that complex situations can arise. It is possible that, in some circumstances, the rights of one patient may conflict with those of another; it may be necessary to spend additional time with one patient to ensure that he or she does not come to any harm, but this means that there is less time to spend with another patient and this may increase that person's risk of harm. Similarly, it is important to recognise that nurses have a duty not only to the patients in their care, but also to their employers, the profession and wider society. They also have a duty of care towards themselves. Again, the potential for competing duties can be seen and this can lead to stress and distress.

> ### Research summary: Violation of ethical principles
>
> Erdil and Korkmaz (2009) undertook a questionnaire survey of 153 nursing students in Turkey. Students were asked five open questions regarding ethical and moral situations they had observed, whether any ethical principles had been violated, the factors that contributed to the ethical problems, the decisions taken by nurses in resolving the situations, and their suggestions as to how nurses could participate in ethical decision making. The most commonly reported problem was psychological maltreatment (34 per cent) followed by inappropriate information (25 per cent) and ignoring patient privacy (24 per cent). The most frequently violated ethical principles were respect for autonomy (30 per cent), respect for privacy and intimacy (22 per cent), the principle of doing no harm (16 per cent), beneficence (17 per cent) and justice (15 per cent). Problems contributing to the ethical problems included the unprofessional behaviour of other professionals, hospital management and inefficient communication. Most students (77 per cent) felt that nurses did not take part in resolving the ethical problems they had observed.

While the research by Erdil and Korkmaz (2009) was undertaken in Turkey, our experience is that similar ethical problems are experienced by nurses working in other countries. It is, therefore, important to understand the nature of such problems and to develop strategies for resolving them.

Ethical dilemmas

The previous section demonstrated how situations can occur where one ethical principle seems to contradict another in certain circumstances. Indeed, it is common to talk of ethical dilemmas. These have been defined as situations in which individuals have to choose between two actions, neither of which is desirable, or situations where it appears impossible to resolve a clash of principles or duties, and there are no clear rules to guide actions (Thompson et al., 2006). Beauchamp and Childress (2009) similarly define such dilemmas as situations in which moral obligations seem to require that an individual perform two or more incompatible actions. Such dilemmas can occur frequently within nursing practice. Take some time to complete Activity 3.6 and think about a dilemma you have encountered.

Activity 3.6   *Reflection*

Think about your own practice and try to identify situations where you felt there was an ethical dilemma.

*   For whom was it a dilemma?
*   What was the basis of the dilemma?
*   How was the dilemma resolved?

Some outline answers are given at the end of the chapter.

Seeking to safeguard patients and clients can give rise to a number of ethical dilemmas. For example, Whitelock (2009), talking about the situation in mental health services, highlights the tension between respecting people's autonomy and the need to provide protection. This challenge is clearly illustrated in the research reported in Whitelock's paper, where 84 people with mental health problems participated in a survey. Eighty-six per cent of respondents indicated that they felt they were responsible for keeping themselves safe, compared with 55 per cent who felt that health professionals were responsible for keeping them safe. The difficulties of balancing personal autonomy with mental health services' need to manage risk is similarly highlighted by Mind (2007), which identifies a further ethical dilemma, in which reducing the risk for one group of people may restrict the autonomy of another group.

Dilemmas can also arise in relation to end-of-life care, where the family may have one view as to whether or not resuscitation should be attempted, while the medical team has another. There are also reports of Do Not Attempt Resuscitation (DNAR) orders being placed on patients' files without the knowledge of the patient's family (Patients Association, 2011; Mencap, 2012). While, in emergency situations, such decisions may have to be made without reference to the family, the ethics of not involving the family in other circumstances should be questioned. The potential for decisions to be made in a discriminatory manner (for example, due to age, disability or perceived quality of life) also needs to be recognised. Having sufficient safeguards in place to address such potential is essential and decisions made need to be carefully justified.

In some instances the individuals concerned may be so ill that they are not able to participate in discussions concerning their end-of-life plans, but there have been recent high-profile cases where individuals have fought legal battles for the right to die. Currently within the United Kingdom it is illegal for anyone to assist another to die, yet nurses may find themselves in a situation in which a critically ill patient is asking for such assistance. Nurses may also feel that they have some sympathy with the views of the patient and thus find themselves in an ethical dilemma. In one sense the action (or lack of action) they need to take is clear, since the legal position forbids providing such assistance. Nonetheless, a nurse may still feel a sense of ethical and moral distress. This situation also illustrates how differing perspectives need to be considered in the context of ethical dilemmas. Sanders and Chaloner (2007) question whether an autonomous patient does have the right to request assistance to die, since he or she must also respect the autonomy of those who provide the care.

Nurse managers may also face ethical dilemmas as they seek to reconcile different pressures and demands. Toren and Wagner (2010) note that nurse managers have a responsibility to promote a safe and ethical environment, within which nurses are able to provide quality care. They thus have responsibilities to both patients and staff, and sometimes these may seem to be conflicting. Furthermore, it must also be remembered that these responsibilities also occur within the context of the wider healthcare organisation, and this may impose another layer of demands upon the manager. Take time to read through the case study below to see how these dilemmas can occur in practice.

Case study: An ethical dilemma for management

Jane Lewis is a ward manager for a medical ward. The ward specialises in caring for men with respiratory problems, but increasingly they are finding that they have a mix of patients. At present all 25 beds are occupied, and Jane has been told that another patient is waiting in A&E to be admitted. As a result of this she has been told that she must discharge one patient, Mr Soames.

Mr Soames lives alone, and even though he is much better than he was on admission, his named nurse (Susan Parr) is concerned that, if he is discharged home, without a proper package of care being in place, he will be at risk. In particular, she is concerned that if he goes home he will not be able to self-care in relation to his hygiene and nutritional needs, and will be at risk of falling. Susan has told Jane about her concerns and Jane now feels torn between her responsibilities in relation to Mr Soames, and her responsibilities to the patient who is waiting in A&E.

Jane decides that it isn't possible to discharge Mr Soames and telephones the bed manager to inform her of this decision. She also explains why this is the case. However, she is then told that Mr Soames will be transferred to another ward, and that her ward must take the new admission. While Jane is still concerned at the disruption this will cause to Mr Soames, she agrees.

The new admission is Mr Wilson, who has respiratory problems. However, he is also very confused and agitated. Jane admits him, settles him into a bed and introduces him to other patients and his nurses. Within a short period of time he gets out of bed, goes to the patient in the bed next to him and starts hitting him,

continued . . .

accusing him of taking his clothes. Jane and Susan go to him, try to calm him and return him to his bed. Understandably the other patient, and his visitors, are also very upset by this incident and need reassurance. The ward staffing level is about to drop as two members of staff are due to go off duty, and Jane has been told that there is no money to bring in agency staff. Nonetheless, she feels that she has to allocate one member of staff to Mr Wilson, for at least the next few hours, until they have a clearer understanding of his needs. Also, there are safety issues in relation to both Mr Wilson and the other patients. Again she feels in a dilemma – should she allocate a member of staff knowing that this will leave the rest of the ward running a nurse short, or should she try to persuade one of the nurses to stay on to work some extra hours? Alternatively, should she go ahead and request an additional member of staff?

Activity 3.7   *Leadership and management*

Think about the case study above and the dilemmas that arose.

- Do you feel Jane acted appropriately?
- What would you do differently?
- How would you respond to the final dilemma?
- What rationale would you provide for your actions?

When you have completed this activity compare your ideas to the outline answers given at the end of the chapter.

Nursing can be a stressful occupation and dealing with ethical dilemmas can increase the level of stress (Erdil and Korkmaz, 2009). Since such conflicts and dilemmas cannot entirely be prevented (Pavlish et al., 2011), taking a systematic approach to addressing such dilemmas is helpful. Frameworks to assist ethical decision making can therefore provide structure to the process, and assist in providing a rationale for action, previously identified as important in the context of ethical practice.

Ethical decision making

This chapter has highlighted how ethical problems and dilemmas can occur in everyday practice. It has also identified that being able to provide a rationale for decisions taken is an important element of ethical practice. To assist us in this process a number of ethical decision-making tools are available, and a review of these will show some common elements relating to assessing the situation, considering alternative approaches and evaluating actions taken. For the purpose of this book these elements are used to provide an ethical decision-making framework that reminds us specifically to remember safeguarding issues. This framework has five key elements (see Figure 3.1) and may be remembered by using the word 'GUARD':

- **G**athering information;
- **U**nderstanding the situation;
- **A**ssessing alternative courses of action and identifying a response;
- **R**esponding using an appropriate strategy;
- **D**etermining the effectiveness.

Each of these stages will be discussed in turn, drawing upon information previously discussed in this chapter.

When confronted with an ethical dilemma there can be a tendency to rush in and to try to resolve it, without fully exploring what the central issues are. Unless it is an emergency situation it is important to first *gather* information as to the nature of the problem or issue, for example: Why is it a problem? Who is it a problem for? What values and principles are involved? Are there any guidelines, codes of practice or policies to assist your decision making? Are there any legal implications?

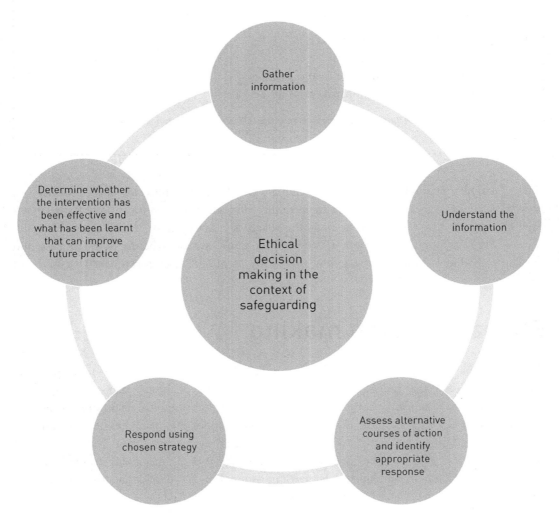

Figure 3.1 Framework for ethical decision making

Having gathered this information it is then necessary to *understand* its significance. For example, it may be that, having looked at the information, there is no longer a dilemma concerning what action to take, as is the case when there is a law or policy that sets out what must be done. Alternatively, it is possible that, having investigated it further, the problem is not as you first understood it. This could occur when previously you only had one person's view of the issue, but now you have other perspectives that provide a different view. At this stage you may also need to consider whether it is necessary to give more weight to one principle or value than another; is it more important to keep someone safe than it is to respect his or her autonomy?

By this stage you should be in a position to *assess* alternative courses of action, taking into account the possible consequences of taking one course in preference to another. Also, the implications of not acting need to be considered. By systematically reviewing these alternatives it should be possible to arrive at a preferred action plan and also to provide a rationale for why you intend to follow a particular course.

When you are *responding* using your chosen course of action, it is important to remain alert to changing situations and the emergence of new issues and information. In some instances this could mean that you need to rethink your strategy and perhaps follow a different course. For example, it could be that you are supporting an older person who is in the early stages of dementia. It had been jointly agreed that the person would continue to manage his or her own affairs for as long as possible and this was the approach being used. However, recently it became apparent that memory loss was becoming a problem and that it could present a risk to personal safety. A reconsideration of approach is thus required. If this is the case, it is once again important to be clear as to why the change was needed.

The final stage encourages you to *determine* whether the approach or intervention has been effective. Here, it is important to consider who should be involved in deciding whether effectiveness has been achieved; a professional view of effectiveness may be different from that of the patient and his or her family. Even if these perspectives differ, however, it is possible to learn from this situation as it can encourage us to reflect critically on our own values and beliefs. Such reflection is essential if ethical practice is to be achieved.

It should be noted that this framework is presented as a circle rather than as a linear process. This is because the process of ethical decision making is an ongoing one. We are constantly learning and developing, and we must recognise the importance of learning from both positive and negative experiences. We often reflect on situations that we feel could have gone better and it is important that we continue to do this. When situations go well we are less likely to reflect upon them and this means that important learning may be lost. Why did things work well? What can we learn from this situation that we can use in future situations? We need to remain open to new learning.

This framework can be used by individuals to provide a basis for considering and responding to ethical dilemmas they encounter, and for developing a sound rationale for actions taken. It could also be used by healthcare teams to determine how best to respond to situations that arise. In the team context, interaction with colleagues who, in some instances, may come from different professional backgrounds can potentially enhance the quality of decision making. Finally, if we are committed to promoting the autonomy of patients and clients, this framework could be used to structure joint decision making between nurses and patients/clients.

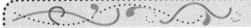

Chapter summary

Seedhouse (2009) argues that ethics is not something that we can be experts in. However, Pavlish et al. (2011) suggest that strengthening nurses' moral reasoning is important. To this end this chapter has explored different ethical perspectives, principles and values. It has also considered the nature of ethical dilemmas and suggested a framework for ethical decision making. Given the ethical dilemmas that can occur in relation to safeguarding adults, the need to strengthen our ethical decision making must be a priority to ensure that our patients and clients are supported in an ethical manner and their interests are safeguarded.

Activities: Brief outline answers

Activity 3.1 Reflection, page 44

As you were asked to identify your personal values, the answer you gave will inevitably be individual to you. However, it is likely that you may have identified some values that many people who choose to be nurses feel are important. These could include values such as respecting people, being non-judgemental, a desire to contribute to society, a belief that people should be supported to achieve their own personal health potential and a view that harming other people is wrong. Such values may influence your desire to become a nurse as you want to help people, to promote health and to protect them from harm. You might feel that you bring personal attributes such as commitment, dedication and enthusiasm to the role. You may have found, however, that some of your values have changed as a result of your nursing experience. For example, working with people from other cultures may make you more aware of different cultural values, which then lead you to re-examine your personal values and beliefs.

Activity 3.2 Critical thinking, page 47

We may be motivated to act by a range of different factors, but when considering this from an ethical perspective we may identify factors such as a sense of duty, respect for other persons or a feeling that injustice is occurring. How we act may be influenced by our personal characteristics (for example, whether we are honest and trustworthy), by the behaviour of those around us (for example, if we feel pressured to conform to the views and behaviours of others), or by predetermined requirements (such as professional codes, policies or legislation). Our behaviour might also be influenced by what we feel will be the consequences of us acting in a particular way or by deciding not to act. We might wish to achieve the maximum benefit for as many people as possible, or we may wish to ensure that one person gains the most, perhaps to correct some form of disadvantage. We may aim to act so as to achieve the outcome that is most fair or just, or we may be in a position where we have to decide which of two alternatives will cause least harm.

Activity 3.3 Decision making and communication, page 48

This is an extremely difficult situation but one that could easily occur. It would be easy to be flattered by the fact that someone feels he or she can trust you enough to confide in you about something extremely difficult. However, it is important to remember that while, as nurses, we would normally aim to promote patient/client autonomy and respect confidentiality, there are some situations in which concerns for an individual's safety have to take precedence: the principle of non-maleficence would need to override that of autonomy.

Activity 3.4 Decision making and communication, page 49

In considering this case study you might have wanted to examine why Mr Holmes becomes aggressive at mealtimes and spits out his food. The staff seem to think this is part of his condition, but did you consider whether Mr Holmes might be trying to communicate by his behaviour. Could it perhaps be his only way of telling them that he doesn't like his food? This may not be the answer, but it could be worth experimenting to see whether different food might change his behaviour. It would seem that Mr Holmes previously valued his autonomy, and to be in a position where he has very limited control over what happens to him must be extremely frustrating. It is also important to note that he has a friend who is visiting him and the staff could work with him to build up a picture of Mr Holmes's personal history, his likes and dislikes and his previously expressed views. Staff could then use this information to provide more personal care and hopefully meet Mr Holmes's needs in the manner he would wish.

Activity 3.5 Critical thinking, page 51

Taken at face value, the phrase 'we treat everybody the same' might be viewed as positive: it could mean that people are not discriminated against in a negative manner. However, where people have additional needs, simply providing the same level of support means that they end up receiving a service that is worse than that provided for other people. In Princy's case, this means that, if 'standard care' is provided, her need for additional support in relation to her posture, communication and health will not be met and she could suffer. The provision of additional support can therefore be justified on the grounds of both non-maleficence (preventing harm) and justice (fairness). In addition, her communication needs mean that it can be difficult for her to exercise any autonomy and other people may act inappropriately in what they believe to be her best interests.

Activity 3.6 Reflection, page 53

In undertaking this activity you may have considered a dilemma that arose due to a clash between your personal values and your professional values, or between your personal values and those of a patient or client. Another source of dilemmas can be the uncertainty that can arise when you feel unsure as to the 'right' way to respond in a situation. This reinforces the need to develop our ethical awareness and our skills in relation to ethical decision making.

Activity 3.7 Leadership and management, page 55

In this case study Jane is confronted by a series of dilemmas. First, there is the dilemma between her concerns for Mr Soames's safety were he to be discharged, and her duty to the patient who is currently waiting in A&E. Jane expresses her concerns and an alternative course of action is put forward. This seems to reduce the potential for harm to Mr Soames while also offering potential benefits for the new patient. However, once this plan is put into practice further dilemmas arise due to the needs of the new patient and the limited availability of staffing. Here Jane, as a manager, is confronted with the competing demands of her responsibilities to keep all patients and staff safe while working in the context of restricted resources. She also feels the need to consider whether she can ask staff to work additional time. The ethical principles of beneficence, non-maleficence and justice are all relevant in this context. In determining what actions Jane might take, you might also consider whether Jane might use her professional autonomy and request additional staff, providing a sound justification for her request based upon ethical principles and concerns regarding the potential consequences should action not be taken. Finally, it is important to remember that Jane has a professional responsibility to maintain the safety of those in her care and to put in writing her concerns if she feels that problems in the care environment are putting others at risk (NMC, 2008a).

Further reading

Fry, ST and Johnstone, M (2008) *Ethics in Nursing Practice: A guide to ethical decision making*, 3rd edition. Oxford: Blackwell.

As the title suggests this book aims to promote ethical decision making. This is achieved through exploration of the responsibilities of nurses and the implications for practice.

Thompson, IE, Melia, KM, Boyd, KM and Horsburgh, D (2006) *Nursing Ethics*, 5th edition. Edinburgh: Churchill Livingstone.

This is a helpful text that addresses both the different approaches to ethics and their application within the context of nursing practice, research, management and education.

Yeo, M, Moorhouse, A, Khan, P and Rodney, P (eds) (2010) *Concepts and Cases in Nursing Ethics*, 3rd edition. Ontario: Broadview Press.

The authors of this text are Canadian and some of the content relates specifically to current challenges in Canada. However, this provides us with a useful comparison and the book also includes discussion of issues, such as truthfulness and integrity, that are not always explored in books concerning nursing ethics.

You may also find it helpful to consult the journal *Nursing Ethics*. This is a journal that focuses solely on ethical aspects of nursing and that publishes both theoretical papers and papers that explore the implications of ethics in nursing practice and education.

Useful websites

www.ethics-network.org.uk

This is the website of the UK Clinical Ethics Network and provides information concerning a range of ethical issues.

www.ethox.org.uk

The Ethox Centre provides support to health professionals regarding clinical and research ethics.

www.icn.ch

This is the website of the International Council of Nurses where you can access its code of ethics.

www.nmc-uk.org

The website of the Nursing and Midwifery Council provides access to all of its documents and standards.

www.nursingethics.ca

This is a Canadian website that provides access to both Canadian and international information concerning nursing ethics.

Chapter 4
Abuse and neglect

continued . . .

19. People can trust the newly registered graduate nurse to work to prevent and resolve conflict and maintain a safe environment.

Cluster: Nutrition and fluid management

28. People can trust the newly registered graduate nurse to assess and monitor their nutritional status and, in partnership, formulate an effective plan of care.

29. People can trust a newly registered graduate nurse to assess and monitor their fluid status and in partnership with them, formulate an effective plan of care.

Chapter aims

After reading this chapter, you will be able to:

- discuss what is meant by the term abuse and the difficulties of developing a suitable definition;
- identify the different types or categories of abuse and the effects it may have on the individual;
- discuss the implications for professional practice.

Introduction

The concept of abuse can be difficult to explain as there are many different forms, types and categories that it can take. Some definitions of abuse can be wide ranging, while others are more focused on specific areas such as particular motivations. The scale of abuse of vulnerable adults is difficult to determine as there are practical and methodological difficulties in researching its incidence (see Chapter 10). Therefore, the aims of this chapter are to develop an understanding of the different forms of abuse and neglect, to explore critically the difficulties with obtaining accurate information concerning incidence and, finally, to understand the effects of abuse and the need for support for an individual who has experienced abuse. First take some time to complete Activity 4.1.

Activity 4.1   *Reflection*

Before we can explore the concept of abuse, it is useful to reflect on what is good practice in order to be able to judge poor and abusive practice. So, for the acronym below, give a term that captures the essential ingredients of a nurse demonstrating good practice. For example, for R you could put 'Respectful'.

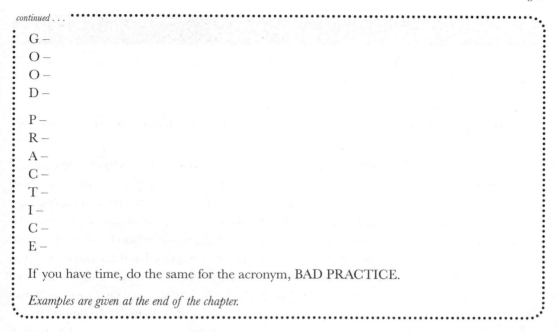

continued . . .

G –

O –

O –

D –

P –

R –

A –

C –

T –

I –

C –

E –

If you have time, do the same for the acronym, BAD PRACTICE.

Examples are given at the end of the chapter.

Much of this text is concerned with the title of an old spaghetti western – *The Good, the Bad and the Ugly*. In Chapter 1, we started off by discussing the good elements of nursing; you may have used some of the main elements of nursing to influence your thoughts in order to address the above reflective activity. We will now address the ugly (abuse) side of practice.

What is abuse?

'Abuse' is a fairly common term used in healthcare to denote an unwelcome activity. Most people would feel that they had some idea of what the term meant and would probably be able to come up with some examples of abuse. It is important for nurses to have a clear understanding of what constitutes abuse. However, it is a very complex issue with many misunderstandings and dilemmas. The first is trying to define the concept. There are a number of different definitions of abuse and most follow the same key principles but vary in the level of detail they provide. The most widely used definition of abuse is provided in both the Department of Health (2000a) document *No Secrets* and in the National Assembly for Wales (2000) document *In Safe Hands*:

Abuse is a violation of an individual's human and civil rights by another person or persons.

Although definitions may vary, they all imply an exertion of one person's power over another (Jenkins and Davies, 2004). This is acknowledged by the following definition provided by the NMC:

Abuse within the practitioner–client relationship is the result of the misuse of power or a betrayal of trust, respect or intimacy between the practitioner and the client, which the practitioner should know would cause physical or emotional harm to the client.
(2002, p5)

Consider the above definitions of abuse. Compare and contrast the relative merits of both and decide which one is more suited to nursing.

Continue reading for suggestions concerning this activity.

The first definition is rather wide ranging and could encompass a range of acts of abuse against a number of people. If you have a wide-ranging definition, you are likely to include and record more abuse taking place. The second definition is narrower in the sense that it focuses specifically on the nurse–client relationship. It also highlights the likely impact of the misuse of power on the client such as physical and emotional harm. The more specific the definition becomes, the more likely it is to exclude acts or actions from being abusive. For example, what if the abuse occurred outside the practitioner–client relationship and/or did not involve a misuse of power? This can be seen with relatives not caring for the client properly due to ignorance or their own problems. How would you be able to assess emotional harm if the client was unable to communicate verbally? Alternatively, having a more specific definition would give you a clearer idea of what constituted abuse. The first wide-ranging definition offers the nurse no direction other than that abuse is a violation of an individual's **civil** and **human rights**, which is open to wide interpretation. Interestingly, the review of *No Secrets* (DH, 2009b) highlighted that there was considerable support for amendment of the current definition used to define abuse. (Human rights and the review of *No Secrets* will be covered in more detail in Chapter 6 on legal and policy provisions.)

Types or categories of abuse

There are a number of well-established categories of abuse (DH, 2000a; NAfW, 2000; Jenkins and Davies, 2004; White, 2011), which cover the following areas.

- *Physical abuse* – This type of abuse involves all forms of physical violence such as hitting, slapping, pushing or kicking. It can also include making people do things against their will, such as eating, bathing and dressing where excessive force is used. Some definitions also include over- or misuse of medication or undue or excessively severe forms of physical restraint. This type of abuse is particularly problematic in the care given to older people and to those with learning disabilities or mental health problems.
- *Sexual abuse* – All definitions of sexual abuse cover severe sexual incidents such as rape or non-consensual sexual assault. Other examples include **buggery**, **incest** and where the perpetrator touches sensitive areas of the body – the genital area, breasts and bottom. This category can also include coercing or encouraging vulnerable people to participate in or watch pornographic material.
- *Psychological abuse* – This is sometimes referred to as emotional abuse and may be intentional or unintentional. It includes insults, threats of harm or abandonment, isolation, deprivation of contact, humiliation, **harassment**, bullying, **persecution**, controlling, intimidation,

withdrawal from services or supportive networks, **coercion** and active denial of rights. There may be more disputes with this type of abuse as it is a particularly subjective category and overlap exists with all other abuse forms. In most forms of abuse there are likely to be psychological or emotional consequences.

- *Financial/material abuse* – This includes financial crimes such as theft or fraud and also exploitation, inappropriate use or misappropriation of a person's financial resources, property, inheritance, pension, allowances or insurance. This type of abuse may also include acts of omission, such as not providing information on benefits to which the vulnerable adult is entitled. Older people may be particularly at risk of this type of abuse.
- *Neglect and acts of omission* – This type of abuse involves the withholding of basic forms of care and necessities of life, resulting in malnutrition, dehydration, poor hygiene, isolation, sleep deprivation, pressure sores etc. There is some overlap with some forms of physical abuse. Pritchard (2001) argues that there are different forms of neglect such as passive and active. In *passive neglect* there is a refusal or failure to act in undertaking necessary care duties. This can include a failure by professionals to access appropriate healthcare on behalf of clients. In *active neglect* there is an intentional act to withhold basic items or resources necessary for safe living. This includes such things as not giving adequate food and drink to clients.

Activity 4.3   *Reflection*

Consider the above categories of abuse and relate them to your current area of practice.

- Do you think they cover all potential areas of abuse?
- If not, what other categories do you feel need to be included?

As this activity concerns your own practice, there is no outline answer at the end of the chapter.

Most national and local policies on abuse will contain the above five main categories of abuse. Recently, many have developed new categories of abuse that focus on the following areas.

- **Discriminatory abuse** – This type of abuse is motivated by discriminatory attitudes in areas such as gender, race, sexual orientation, disability, religion and culture. There is also specific employment legislation that covers these areas and offers some redress to individuals if they feel that they have been discriminated against in the workplace.
- **Institutional abuse** – The recent review of *In Safe Hands* (the Welsh policy guidance document) recommended that institutional abuse (discussed in Chapter 1) should be added as a distinct category in the revised guidance (Magill et al., 2010).

Incidence of abuse

Before reading on, complete Activity 4.4.

The incidence of abuse is determined from two main sources of information: official statistics of reported abuse and research studies (some of which use these official statistics). Both of these sources have their limitations and the difficulties in gathering these data are discussed further in Chapter 10. However, to give you some level of understanding of the incidence of abuse two studies are reported here.

Research summary: The incidence of abuse

O'Keeffe et al. (2007) undertook a UK study of abuse of older people aged 66+ years living in private households, and found that 2.6 per cent of people reported that they had experienced mistreatment involving a family member, close friend or care worker during the past year. They estimate that this would mean that approximately 227,000 older people were neglected or abused in the past year in the UK. The incidence for each type of abuse can be seen in Table 4.1.

Type of abuse	Incidence
Neglect	1.1% or 11 people in 1,000
Financial	0.7% or 7 people in 1,000
Psychological	0.4% or 4 people in 1,000
Physical	0.4% or 4 people in 1,000
Sexual	0.2% or 2 people in 1,000
Combination of 2 types of abuse	6%

Table 4.1 Types and incidence of abuse (O'Keeffe et al., 2007)

Beadle-Brown et al. (2010) explored the nature of adult protection referrals made between the years 1998 and 2005 from two local authorities in the southeast of England. The study was primarily aimed at exploring the abuse of people with learning disabilities, but it also compared data with other vulnerable groups (see Table 4.2). The total number of cases was 6,148, of which 1,926 referred to people with learning disabilities.

Type of abuse	People with learning disabilities (%)	Other vulnerable groups (%)
Multiple types of abuse	33	29.8
Sexual	17.3	3.1
Physical	28.9	21.7
Psychological	6.1	6.7
Financial	7.2	17.8
Institutional	1.4	4.4
Discriminatory	0.1	0.2
Neglect	5.5	16
Other	0.5	0.2
Where abuse took place		
Residential care	55.7	52.1
Own home	19.1	41.6
Day care setting	5.6	0.3
Health setting	2.1	1.7
Public place	7.2	0.7
Other	8.3	3.6
Type of abuser		
Service user	26.4	6.4
Family/partner/carer	23.3	39.9
Manager/owner	9.3	8.5
All types of staff	37.2	42.3
Health worker	0.5	0.7
Other	3.4	2.2

Table 4.2 Referrals by types of abuse (Beadle-Brown et al., 2010)

Neglect

It would be fair to say that neglect is the neglected area when exploring types of abuse. This is surprising as neglect is an element of most cases of abuse, particularly institutional abuse. Practitioners can be confused about what exactly constitutes this form of abuse and one study found that they rarely described neglect as a form of abuse (Taylor and Dodd, 2003). It has already been highlighted, when we explored the different types of abuse above, that there are two different types of neglect – active and passive. The first is often perceived as more severe as there is an element of intent by the abuser, and the latter is somehow less severe as the abuser did not intend for the abuse to occur. Regardless of the intentions of the care giver, the potential impact and harm may be the same for the patient/client. A major difficulty in addressing the issue of neglect is that it can often be difficult to detect or prove that it has happened. To understand the implications of this, take some time to complete Activity 4.5.

Activity 4.5   *Critical thinking*

- Consider the following case scenarios and determine whether you feel the neglect is active or passive.
- Why do you think it may be difficult to prove that neglect has happened?

Scenario 1: Jane Howells is a 31-year-old woman with severe learning disabilities. She has been admitted to hospital for tests as her mother insists she is not well. Jane has started to refuse food and drink and will not let staff near her to carry out tests as she is reluctant to let people touch her. She was sexually abused in the past and the medical opinion is that her problems might be more psychological than physical, although her mother is not happy with this. The medical team wants to discharge her home, although Jane has had very little food and drink for the week she has been in hospital.

Scenario 2: Tom Harris is an 82-year-old man who has been admitted to a private nursing home as he can no longer care for himself and is in the early stages of dementia. He was a former university professor and likes to read *The Times* newspaper every morning. He identified this in his care plan as well as the impact if he missed a day. On two occasions in the last month the staff have failed to provide the newspaper for him, much to his annoyance. Tom's son has complained to the lead nurse who replied, 'For goodness sake, I have more important things to worry about than a few missing newspapers.'

Scenario 3: Mary James is a 42-year-old woman who has had a series of depressive episodes for the last 20 years and is also addicted to cannabis. At times she is reluctant to leave her ground-floor flat and keeps a number of cats and other pets. She does not let her pets out and keeps them locked up all day. She very rarely changes her clothes, does not eat very much and is reluctant to throw away any waste. Her community mental health nurse monitors her situation and her compliance with medication. She has had previous admissions for severe depression and for being at risk. Her neighbour in the flat above is not happy with the smell coming from her flat and the piles of newspapers, which he feels pose a serious fire risk.

There are some comments below and an outline answer at the end of the chapter.

In scenario 1, it would appear that this is a case of active neglect as Jane has not received the necessary level of nutrition and fluid you would expect of a patient who has been in the care of professionals for a week. The plan of care seems ineffective in this instance. There is evidence of the known difficulty for vulnerable people in receiving suitable levels of food and drink. This is a particular problem for older people and people with learning disabilities. A headline from the *Daily Mail* (9 January 2009) highlighted the case of *Martin Ryan, a 43 year old man with Down syndrome who starved to death in an NHS hospital when he went without food for 26 days*.

There is also evidence of passive neglect in this scenario as Jane may be being denied access to appropriate healthcare. In the past it could be claimed that health staff were not fully aware of the health needs and difficulties that people with learning disabilities may face in accessing appropriate healthcare. However, as the evidence is widely available and has been around for many years, this defence is very questionable. In terms of detecting neglect, you can understand the difficulties faced here. It would be straightforward if the records had been kept up to date with regard to fluid and nutritional intakes during the week she was in hospital. If a baseline assessment had been done on the first day, you would be able to tell if she had lost any weight. Other tests would reveal if she was malnourished and dehydrated or not. However, as she is refusing to eat or drink, obviously this makes things difficult for the nursing staff. If she was discharged home and subsequently it was found that she did have a treatable illness, the hospital is likely to be found negligent and her health needs have been neglected.

Regarding scenario 2, many people may behave like the lead nurse and think it is all a storm in a teacup. However, it must be remembered that, if a service is truly person centred, what is important to the client should be important to the staff. The problem with detecting and proving neglect is that is often not a single event. Neglect is seen as a series of failures to provide basic care or items. Action on Elder Abuse (2012) disagree with academics and feel that just one incident can be severe in terms of impact and neglect should never be underestimated. In this case, would two occasions in a month be sufficient to say that Tom's needs were being neglected? What if we were to look at two occasions in six months? Were the papers not provided intentionally (active) or had a nurse simply forgotten or thought they were not important enough (passive)? The reaction of the lead nurse would indicate that providing newspapers was not important enough. In terms of the impact on Tom, would he really be abused by missing two days' papers? As a paying customer, he is not receiving what he has paid for and the service is failing him. In the past, neglect tended to focus too much on the physical impact rather than social and psychological needs. Tom is clearly annoyed and, as he has early-stage dementia, maintaining routines and familiar events and behaviours should be part of the overall care package. Therefore, there may well be a psychological impact on Tom.

Finally, in scenario 3 there is evidence of self-neglect, whereby the client is seen to neglect his or her own needs by the life choices made. This is a complex area of practice for the community nurse, with a balance of respecting Mary's autonomy while ensuring that her health and well-being are not made worse. Most safeguarding policies and procedures tend not to include self-neglect as there is not another person (abuser) involved (Braye et al., 2011). Therefore, there is nobody from whom to safeguard Mary other than herself.

The above scenarios have highlighted some of the difficulties in deciding what active, passive or self-neglect is. In the following case study, we can see the practical difficulties of preventing neglect and in determining if it has occurred or not.

> ### Case study: Pressure sores
>
> *Steven is a 36-year-old man who suffered a spinal cord injury when he came off his mountain bike in the Scottish highlands. He has been on a rehabilitation unit while recovering from his accident. He has lost the use of his legs and has had to come to terms with using a wheelchair. On a recent visit, his mother, who was once a nurse, noticed that he had three grade 2 pressure sores on his legs. She informed the nurse who said that they had been very busy due to staff shortages and increased admissions.*

Many safeguarding policies and procedures include the development of pressure sores as an indicator of neglect. It is very difficult to argue against this and effective nursing practice should always prevent the development of pressure skin damage. It is known that people who have mobility difficulties have susceptibility to this type of damage as they cannot move around and pressure is put on particular parts of the body. Dougherty and Lister (2011) highlight reasons, other than self-neglect, why some patients are more likely to have skin breakdown due to pressure damage:

- poor health status of the patient or degenerative conditions;
- poor nutritional and fluid intake;
- neurological disorders;
- side effects of some medication;
- certain blood disorders;
- **ischaemia**;
- accidents or unexpected incidents.

If we take the view that pressure sores are not inevitable and are preventable, the development of such a health problem must be down to the neglect of staff caring for the client. Some staff may use a variety of reasons for this happening, such as shortage of staff, not enough time, lack of training, someone else's responsibility or not enough lifting equipment, or they may blame the patient for being uncooperative or some other factor such as the patient being over- or underweight. These reasons may make things more difficult, but again tissue damage due to pressure is preventable. Nurses can enlist the help of patients and promote self-help in order to minimise the chances of pressure sores developing.

Thresholds and decision making

It was highlighted in Chapter 1 that some nurses will speak out and report suspected abuse while others remain silent. As nurses have a duty to speak out, such silence may be viewed as consent to the abusive act taking place (Nazarko, 2001). However, it is not always clear if abuse has actually taken place. One of the difficulties is that there is very little guidance on 'thresholds for action'. That is, at what point does a nurse take action if he or she suspects abuse has taken place? The idea that 'thresholds for action' are important is just beginning to be recognised (Jenkins et al., 2008; Collins, 2010), as we try to understand why there is not consistency in dealing with abuse and how decisions are arrived at by professionals such as nurses. One of the factors that may influence nurses in deciding whether to take action or not is the existence of a '**hierarchy of abuse**'. Jenkins et al.'s (2008) study supported this notion, as staff were very clear that they would act if sexual or physical abuse was taking place. However, there was less certainty about other types of abuse, particularly neglect, which was largely ignored. Interestingly, participants in this study also felt that client-on-client abuse was less severe than staff-on-client abuse.

Activity 4.6   *Critical thinking*

- In terms of a hierarchy of abuse, what sorts of factors would nurses use to 'weigh up' whether they would act on abuse or not?
- Consider the hierarchy of abuse in Figure 4.1. In what order, in terms of severity or seriousness, would you rank the different types of abuse?

Continue reading the text for comments on this activity.

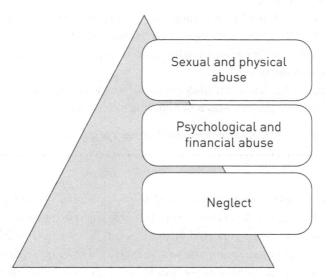

Figure 4.1 Hierarchy of abuse

In Figure 4.1 it is clear that sexual and physical abuse are at the top. This may be because these types of abuse are generally viewed as being the most severe or have the greatest impact not only on the victim, but also on those who witness such events. They are very traumatic for all those involved, for example rape cases or someone being punched or kicked unconscious. These types of cases may pose fewer problems when it comes to gathering evidence for possible prosecutions. DNA testing of semen can determine if intercourse has taken place if a condom was not worn, and bruising from a punch can also be powerful evidence. Financial abuse may be less troublesome to prove as good accounting procedures and record keeping can point the finger at the potential culprit. This type of abuse may be viewed as less serious if the victim is rich or careless with money. Psychological abuse is less visible when the victim is unable or unwilling to display his or her hurt behaviour through actions. You are often left waiting for the victim to describe how he or she feels if the person is able to talk about it. People can be so traumatised they are unable to speak about the abuse, or they bury it deep into their unconscious and may act as if nothing has happened. Therefore, if there are no outward signs, it is not surprising for others to feel there has been minimal impact. Neglect is usually seen at the bottom of the list for the reasons discussed above in the section on neglect.

Activity 4.7   *Reflection and critical thinking*

Consider the following situations and decide when and if you would take action. You will also need to decide if there is evidence of bad practice or abuse. Once you have made up your mind for the five situations, consult with your colleagues and get their views.

1. Forgetting to put out a clean towel for a patient for one day and not changing the sheets for three days.
2. Not including the patient's views, or those of his or her carer/family, when undertaking a person-centred care plan.
3. A fellow nurse who is a relative confides in you that he has given the wrong drug to a patient, but it is all right as nothing serious has happened.
4. You are on your own with a patient who grabs your private parts and you instantly slap the person across the face.
5. A fellow nurse, who has been under a lot of stress recently due to losing both his children, swears at a patient who is demanding to have the ward television in his room.

For comments on situation 1, read on; there are outline answers to situations 2–5 at the end of the chapter.

These five situations should demonstrate some of the complexities of working in healthcare and the thresholds for deciding to take action or not. If a zero tolerance to abuse is in operation, you would expect all five cases to be reported at some point. Nurses may weigh up all the factors before deciding, but as an organisation you would expect them to be reported. However, if you explore each one, there would be factors you would take into account before reaching a decision. If we take the first scenario, just forgetting a clean towel on one day or not changing sheets for three days may each be viewed as poor practice. However, taken together they may indicate neglect. It is unlikely that the missing towel would be reported, but the three days of unchanged sheets might, and together they most definitely should be reported. A zero tolerance strategy or good practice guide may set out exactly what a service should provide. So if patients can expect a clean towel and sheets every day, this is the standard that should be met and addressed at the time if these actions are not done.

Hate crime

The following quote from the Dalai Lama illustrates the destructiveness of anger and hatred:

Anger may seem to offer an energetic way of getting things done, but such a perception of the world is misguided. The only certainty about anger and hatred is that they are destructive.

Case study: Hate crime murder

Steven Hoskin was a 38-year-old man with learning disabilities who lived in St Austell, Cornwall, in 2006. He was befriended by a group of people and some of them moved into his bedsit with him. Initially, he received two hours of social care support each week, but later he declined this service and his active case was closed. Over a period of time, the people he thought of as friends started to abuse him and take advantage of living in his flat. One day he was made to wear a dog collar, was burnt with cigarettes and forced to confess he was a paedophile. In the evening he was again abused and forced to swallow a large number of painkillers. He was then taken to a nearby railway viaduct and made to hang on the wrong side of a safety rail. The girlfriend of one of his abusers stood on his hands and he fell to his death, from a height of 30 metres. Steven had a fear of heights. A 29-year-old man and a 16-year-old girl (at the time of his death) were both convicted of Steven's murder in 2007, while another man, aged 21, was convicted of his manslaughter.

The high-profile hate crime murder of Steven Hoskin demonstrated the extreme lengths some people would go to in acting out their **prejudices** or hatred against people whom they viewed as inferior or different. Hate crime has been defined by the Crown Prosecution Service (CPS, 2012a) as *any crime where the perpetrator's hostility or prejudice against an identifiable group of people is a factor in determining who is victimised*. The CPS and the Association of Chief Police Officers (ACPO) have agreed on this definition and focus on five distinct areas: disability, race, religion and belief, sexual orientation and transgender identity. They list some of the many forms of abuse that hate crime can take (see Table 4.3).

The evidence in this case suggests that had Mr Hoskin not been a person with a learning disability, he may not have been murdered. Sadly, this was not a one-off event and is a real threat faced by all people with disabilities. An aspect of this case is that he was befriended by people whom he thought of as friends. This has also been referred to as 'mate crime', whereby members of the wider community develop friendships with vulnerable people in order to exploit and take advantage of them. Some individuals will actively seek out vulnerable individuals, while others take advantage of or create their own opportunities. This can be a particular problem for some groups of people, such as those with learning disabilities, as they often find it difficult to form and maintain friendships (McConkey, 2007). Older people can also be at risk if they live alone and have outlived many of their friends and family members. The types of people who commit hate crime and the number of crimes with conviction rates are given in Figure 4.2.

Type of hate crime	Examples
Physical attacks	• physical assault • damage to property • offensive graffiti • arson
Threat of attack	• offensive letters • abusive or obscene telephone calls • groups hanging around to intimidate • unfounded, malicious complaints
Verbal abuse, insults or harassment	• taunting • offensive leaflets and posters • abusive gestures • dumping of rubbish outside homes or through letterboxes • bullying at school or in the workplace

Table 4.3 Forms of hate crime

The number of hate crimes referred to the CPS has steadily increased from 14,133 in 2006/7 to 15,519 in 2010/11.

The proportion of successful convictions increased from 76.8% in 2006/7 to 82.8% in 2010/11. A guilty plea was offered in 85.5% of successful outcomes.

The majority of perpetrators of hate crimes were white British men aged 25–59 and 28.9% aged 18–24.

Figure 4.2 Hate crime statistics for 2010–11 (CPS, 2012b)

Activity 4.8 — Critical thinking

Consider the issues in the following case study of Charles.

• Do you believe this to be a hate or mate crime or some other form of crime/abuse?
• What are the implications for a registered nurse in this case study?

Comments on this activity are given below and at the end of the chapter.

Case study: Hate crime, mate crime, or something else?

Charles is a 68-year-old man who has had to contend with mania for most of his life. He has no close friends or living family members. He has always had problems forming friendships due to his behaviour and the stigma of his condition. He has a female registered mental health nurse who provides six hours of therapy and support a week for him. She helps him with his medication, interpersonal skills and self-image. She also helps him with his shopping, cooking and cleaning, and sometimes they go to the cinema together in her own time. She is fully aware that she should be supporting and encouraging Charles to be independent, but she finds it easier to do the tasks for him as it saves time. He looks forward to her coming to his house as he enjoys her company.

During a manic episode he hit the nurse but she forgave him and said she would not report the incident. Charles was pleased with this and gave her extra money for shopping to go and buy herself something. Recently, Charles has noticed that his shopping bill has increased and some money from his wallet has gone missing. When he mentioned it to the registered nurse she reminded him of their 'secret' and that he could get into a lot of trouble for hitting her and making false allegations. She explained that she doesn't get much money from the care agency and sometimes needed more cash for her disabled son who sometimes accompanies her when she is working with Charles. Charles said he understood and he would help as much as he could, and told her he would prefer to lend her money rather than have her take it. He even suggested that he could care for her son while she was at work. Charles believes she loves him as she has kissed him passionately several times, but she insists that they could only ever be friends.

This is not a clear-cut case of hate or mate crime, but there are dire consequences for the registered nurse. The nurse, as a member of the public, has not shown hostility or prejudice against Charles. Far from it, she has shown some kindness and some understanding. These are some elements of mate crime in the sense that she has developed a friendship with Charles as part of her role as his nurse and has used it to her own advantage. The real issue here is her abuse of power and unprofessional behaviour. The nurse has used her privileged position to gain the trust of Charles and has then crossed the boundary of the nurse–client relationship. She has crossed this several times in this situation. First, she is maintaining and then developing Charles's dependency on her when she should be doing the opposite by supporting him to remain relatively independent through an empowering process. As a result, her reason for being with Charles becomes unclear to both of them. Second, she fails to report an assault – at best, this does not follow local policy for reporting of such incidents and, at worst, she uses it as a sort of insurance to maintain her control or power over Charles. There is not enough detail in the case study to know if she manipulated the situation in order for Charles to hit her. In Chapter 1, we explored perpetrator motivations, in which some individuals look to exploit or create opportunities in which to abuse others. There may well have been some manipulation in this situation.

The NMC (2009) is very clear with its guidance on sexual boundaries, which has in some ways replaced its previous guidance on practitioner–client relationships and the prevention of abuse (NMC, 2002). Both guidance documents make clear to registered nurses the boundaries and limits of behaviour expected between nurses and their clients. Such relationships should be based on trust, respect and the appropriate use of power and should focus exclusively on the needs of the client. It is always the responsibility of the registered nurse to maintain appropriate professional boundaries. In the above case study it is clear that the nurse has overstepped the boundaries by developing this personal relationship by abusing her power. This is seen by some of her behaviour in passionately kissing the client, seeing Charles outside working hours, bringing her son into his home and developing Charles's dependency on her.

Domestic violence

This type of abuse tends to sit outside safeguarding and adult protection work, and this is reflected in the lack of literature linking it to this area (Mornington and Mornington, 2008).

Domestic violence or abuse is a complex problem and is a worldwide significant health issue (McGarry et al., 2011). It is often a hidden problem and tends to occur behind closed doors in the family home. Domestic Violence (2012) offers a definition of domestic violence as:

> *any incident of threatening behaviour, violence or abuse (psychological, physical, sexual, financial or emotional) between adults, aged 18 and over, who are or have been intimate partners or family members, regardless of gender and sexuality.*

The World Health Organization (WHO, 2005) study on domestic violence undertaken in a number of different countries found that it largely involved women, although all genders are affected. Women were more at risk in the home compared to the street, and abused women were twice as likely compared to non-abused women to have poor physical and mental health problems. Pregnancy posed particular problems and the study found between 4 and 12 per cent of women had reported being beaten. The fathers of the unborn children would be responsible for abusing more than 90 per cent of these women, often by kicking or punching them in the abdomen. In the UK, Women's Aid, a national domestic violence charity for women and children, provides some statistics on domestic abuse (see Figure 4.3).

Activity 4.9   *Critical thinking*

Analyse the statistics in Figure 4.3 and answer the following questions.

- Why does domestic violence seem to focus exclusively on women?
- Why do you think men are not included?
- Why is it difficult to get accurate information?
- Are there any particular cultural differences in the types of domestic violence occurring in the UK?

Answers are provided in the following text.

Domestic violence can occur in a range of relationships including heterosexual, gay, lesbian and transgender relationships.

Less than 50% of all incidents of domestic violence are reported to the police.

1 in 4 women will experience domestic violence in their lifetime.

Women may experience domestic violence regardless of ethnicity, religion, class, age, sexuality, disability or lifestyle.

2 women per week are killed by current or ex-partners.

Figure 4.3 Domestic violence statistics (Women's Aid, 2012)

As highlighted above, evidence strongly suggests that women are at the greatest risk of domestic violence compared to men (WHO, 2005; Mornington and Mornington, 2008). The statistics provided in Figure 4.3 come from the charity Women's Aid, which is for female victims of domestic violence. A report developed by the male campaign group, Parity, claims that abuse by wives and girlfriends is largely ignored by the police and that two in five of all victims of domestic abuse are men (*The Observer*, 2010). Domestic abuse is also seen within gay partnerships. Each group tends to have gender biases, although even the male group's claims suggest that women are more likely to be subject to domestic violence. It is difficult to obtain accurate statistics because domestic violence is a hidden problem. Therefore, there is still a reluctance to report abuse due to feelings of shame, cultural issues, stigma, fear of further abuse and not being believed. Men may feel that others will think they are weak or not proper men if they report that their female partners are abusing them. It is therefore not surprising that some may feel that domestic violence may be under-reported and an even bigger problem than we think.

> ### Case study: Public or private violence?
>
> *Shannon is a 19-year-old woman from the traveller community who has recently been admitted to her local maternity unit. Jayne, a student nurse on placement in the unit, overheard Shannon's husband shouting at her and saw him pulling her hair violently. Shannon explained to Jayne that the husband in her culture is the 'boss' and the wife must be at his beck and call. She said she does not mind the occasional slap as she deserves it and it's not a problem.*

In the above case study, the student nurse may be confused as to what to do in this situation. It may be clear that Shannon does not see that she may have been subjected to domestic violence; after all, she dismisses the incident as part of her life or culture. The student may believe this is permissible as nurses should respect the cultural, spiritual and religious beliefs of those in their care. However, in this instance, an alleged assault has taken place in a public place and as such should not be tolerated. The student nurse should report exactly what she witnessed and also seek guidance from her mentor. If this had taken place at home it is unlikely that Shannon would have reported her husband. This incident highlights the difficulties of domestic violence and illustrates how it can impact on **therapeutic relationships** in the healthcare setting and, as such, be subject to safeguarding procedures. Potentially different rules and behaviours may seem to apply in public and private arenas. Even though such abusive behaviours may be culturally tolerated, they will inevitably fall foul of the laws and codes of behaviour expected of the society in which they take place. There are also issues in the Muslim and south Asian communities with honour-based crimes. In extreme cases, young women have been murdered because it has been felt by relatives or communities that they have brought shame or dishonour on their families by not going along with arranged marriages (Mornington and Mornington, 2008), or by embracing Western values and behaviours.

The effects of abuse

The effects of abuse can be long term and in some cases create a lifetime of personal difficulties for the abused person. In Chapter 1, reference was made to the survivors of the Longcare abuse scandal (see the further reading in that chapter for a full account). John Pring's biography of a care scandal caught up with some of the survivors of the appalling abuse that took place, to see how they survived the abusive regime. He felt that they had shown remarkable resilience and also courage during and since their ordeal. In spite of such courage and resilience, the long-term effects of abuse can have a profound and damaging impact on the individual and their families. It is not only clients who suffer the effects of abuse. Nurses are also subjected to verbal abuse by fellow nurses, particularly by staff nurses. Nurses who are subjected to this type of abuse are more stressed and likely to have poor job satisfaction, taking more time off. Ultimately, these nurses will give poor-quality service to people in their care (Rowe and Sherlock, 2005).

Activity 4.10 | *Reflection*

Imagine the likely short- and long-term impact of abuse for the following areas:

- domestic abuse for older women;
- abuse in childhood on self-esteem;
- abuse of people with severe learning disabilities and their families.

The following research summary will be helpful in completing this activity.

Research summary: The impacts of abuse

McGarry et al. (2011) undertook a review of the literature concerning the impact of domestic abuse on older women. The literature would suggest that it tends to focus on younger women and largely ignores the impact on the older generation because of the blurring between elder abuse and domestic abuse. The impact of domestic abuse on older women was found to take the form of mental health problems such as anxiety and depression, which are likely, in turn, to impact on relationships and levels of support. This then increases the chances of developing physical health problems, possibly leading to premature death.

Sachs-Ericsson et al.'s (2010) large-scale two-part study ($n=1460$ and $n=1090$) found that abuse in childhood can have a lasting effect into old age. They also found that it can have a greater impact on those who already had low self-esteem compared to those with higher levels. Encouragingly, the study also found that some individuals were able to deal with the abuse affecting their self-concept, which therefore reduced the negative impact on their mental health.

O'Callaghan et al.'s (2003) small-scale study ($n=18$) explored the impact of abuse on people with severe learning disabilities and their families. This study also found the impact of abuse to be long lasting for both the victims and their families. The informants of the survivors of abuse reported a variety of symptoms and challenging behaviours. These included self-injury, soiling and a loss of self-help skills and language, with an overall regression in terms of development. The family members of the survivors reported feelings of anger towards services for letting the abuse happen and of guilt for not seeing or stopping the abuse.

Support for people who have been abused

There are two aspects to consider when supporting vulnerable adults who have been abused. The first is supporting the victim after the abuse has taken place and the second is supporting the person through the safeguarding and criminal proceedings to ensure the perpetrator/s are brought to account for their abusive actions. Supporting people after abuse is essential – the previous section highlighted the long-term or lifetime impact of abuse on the survivor. Many individuals who are subjected to traumatic events such as abuse may develop symptoms of post-traumatic stress disorder (PTSD). Access the NHS Choices webpage on www.nhs.uk/ Conditions/Post-traumatic-stress-disorder/Pages/Introduction.aspx for information on the symptoms, causes, diagnosis and treatment of this condition.

Post-abuse support is now focusing and listening more to what survivors of abuse are saying. It can be easy for professionals to sit back and feel they know best when it comes to treatments. It is important for survivors to have both short- and long-term help. Some vulnerable adult survivors of abuse shared their experiences, through group-work sessions, of what was helpful for them. Some found that writing poems, counselling, being listened to and being part of a group helped them come to terms with their experiences. Some survivors found it comforting to find out the truth when abusers had threatened and lied to them to keep their silence (Pritchard, 2008). This area of practice is still developing as professionals listen to the stories of survivors and try to develop innovative therapies and approaches.

The second area of post-abuse support is ensuring survivors are helped through safeguarding and criminal proceedings. More attention is being given to ensuring that vulnerable adults receive justice against those who have abused them (DH, 2009b, 2009c). In the past this was not given a priority and perpetrators would get away with abuse and then go on and abuse further victims until they were stopped.

Activity 4.11   *Critical thinking*

* Consider carefully why ensuring justice was not given a priority.
* Why would it be difficult to prove and secure convictions for perpetrators of abuse against vulnerable adults?

The section on perpetrators of abuse in Chapter 1 (pages 19–21) may be particularly helpful to you in completing this activity. There is no outline answer at the end of the chapter.

Perpetrators of abuse often prey on vulnerable adults as they know that some individuals are unable to speak due to a disability, or that the disability carries such a stigma that, even if they are able to speak, it is unlikely that they will be believed or even listened to. When abuse has been carried out by a carer or family member, this makes it even more difficult for the individual, who is dependent on them for his or her needs. Survivors' stories confirm this in that they were beaten, threatened with more harm and even told that no one would believe them (Pritchard, 2008). The legal system is trying to get to grips with this and now more effort is put into securing convictions by supporting and protecting victims through the process and in giving evidence in court. Specialist teams and the use of technology have helped victims during the legal process. Society is now more aware of abuse scandals that have taken place within a number of our established institutions, such as children's homes and the church. Therefore, people are prepared to think the unthinkable and that vulnerable children and adults can be abused anywhere and by anyone.

Listening to survivors of abuse was the aim of a small-scale qualitative study (*n=4*) by Davies et al. (2009) regarding the experiences of vulnerable adults undertaking the adult-protection process.

The study found that vulnerable adults had little understanding of safeguarding policies and practices, although they felt supported, protected and listened to. However, the Protection of Vulnerable Adults (POVA) process was viewed as potentially very disempowering and the study made the recommendations listed in Box 4.1.

Box 4.1: Recommendations for improving vulnerable adults' experience of undergoing safeguarding procedures (Davies et al., 2009)

- Procedures should be incorporated into policies for actively involving vulnerable adults in investigations (if they want this). Develop specific guidance for vulnerable adult involvement in POVA.
- Communication challenges should not be viewed as a barrier to involvement.
- The safeguarding process should be empowering for the vulnerable adult.
- Share good practice around vulnerable adult involvement in adult protection/safeguarding.
- When a vulnerable adult is the perpetrator this poses specific challenges – consider the time it takes to create safety for both.
- Ideas of justice may differ for vulnerable adults – involve their views wherever possible and at the very least keep them informed about what is happening at each stage.
- Give greater attention to 'outcomes for the victim' – many vulnerable adults want reassurance that the abuse will stop and that some sort of punishment will occur.
- Ongoing protection needs to operate at three levels: victim, other victims and wider safety issues.

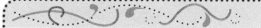

Chapter summary

This chapter has explored the concept of abuse and how definitions can have an impact on the perception of the incidence of abuse. The frequency of abuse can be difficult to determine due to a number of issues, although any abuse perpetrated against vulnerable adults must be a cause for concern. Specific types of abuse may be viewed as more severe than others and efforts have been made to reduce the amount of hate crime against different groups of people. Neglect, in particular, poses many challenges for professionals and services as it can often be difficult to detect. The thresholds for nurses taking action may vary depending on the context, nature of relationships, experience and perceptions of those who witness abuse taking place. Finally, more emphasis needs to be placed on supporting and empowering survivors of abuse.

Activities: Brief outline answers

Activity 4.1 Reflection, pages 62–3

Some examples are:

G – Gracious/good communicator
O – Observant
O – Organised
D – Dignified/diligent/dedicated

P – Person centred/perceptive/passionate
R – Respectful/resourceful/reflective
A – Attentive/approachable/adaptable
C – Caring
T – Team player
I – Insightful
C – Compassionate
E – Emotionally stable/empathetic

Acronyms are useful in terms of memorising aspects of good practice, but they are limited as you have to fit in terms that match the acronym. You would also expect nurses demonstrating good practice to be safe, knowledgeable and have sound judgement. In terms of **BAD PRACTICE**, you may have found this easier to do and this will require further reflection on why this may be the case. A nurse demonstrating such practice may be:

B – Boastful/brash
A – Arrogant
D – Deceitful

P – Patronising
R – Rigid
A – Abusive
C – Crass/clueless
T – Tactless
I – Insensitive/ignorant
C – Callous
E – Emotionless

Activity 4.5 Critical thinking, page 68

Scenario 1: Access the following Mencap documents, which highlight the difficulties that people with learning disabilities face in accessing appropriate healthcare.

Mencap (2004) *Treat Me Right: Better healthcare for people with a learning disability.* London: Mencap.

Mencap (2007) *Death by Indifference: Following up the Treat Me Right report.* London: Mencap.

Mencap (2012) *Death by Indifference: 74 deaths and counting. A progress report 5 years on.* London: Mencap.

The following article discusses how nurses may be held accountable for the neglect of people with learning disabilities by not ensuring access to appropriate healthcare.

Jenkins, R and Davies, R (2006) Neglect of people with intellectual disabilities: A failure to act? *Journal of Intellectual Disabilities*, 10(1): 35–45.

Scenario 3: The following article should help you with the issue of self-neglect as it discusses how it relates to safeguarding.

Braye, S, Orr, D and Preston-Shoot, M (2011) Conceptualising and responding to self-neglect: the challenges for adult safeguarding. *Journal of Adult Protection*, 13(4): 182–93.

Activity 4.7 Reflection and critical thinking, page 72

2. This would be very bad practice bordering on abuse as person-centred care must include the client's views or perspective. The use of an independent advocate would ensure that the voice of the client was respected. All efforts should be used to include the views of carers/families in the care planning process (NMC, 2009).
3. You must act without delay and seek medical advice in the interests of the client. Any loyalties must be set aside and you should, with your fellow nurse, ensure this is done. Mistakes with medication do happen and the consequences for delayed action may be fatal. See further advice on the administration of medication on the NMC website.
4. You should report the incident as well as your actions immediately and any reasonable organisation would take into account all the circumstances. You will need support for this sexual assault as well as the patient. Organisations should be ensuring that staff self-report incidents such as this, encouraging openness and not imposing such harsh sanctions as dismissal, as this will just discourage such self-reporting actions.
5. While you may have a lot of sympathy for this nurse, you should report this verbal abuse immediately so a full investigation can take place. It can then take into account this nurse's personal circumstances when deciding what further action needs to be taken.

Activity 4.8 Critical thinking, page 74

The types of abuse occurring in this case study include financial, psychological and sexual abuse. The nurse may be breaking the Sexual Offences Act 2003 in developing a 'sexual relationship' that results in harm, exploits the individual in her care and therefore undermines public confidence. She is also potentially putting her son at risk by bringing him into work, particularly if she decides to leave him with Charles. This is not because Charles has a psychiatric illness but because it would go against local policy guidance; it is not good practice and it further strengthens the inappropriate relationship that has been developing. It would also potentially invalidate her indemnity insurance if she had cover from her trade union. Further information regarding clear sexual boundaries is obtainable from the NMC at www.nmc-uk.org.

Further reading

Collins, M (2010) Thresholds in adult protection. *Journal of Adult Protection*, 12(1): 4–12.

This is a useful article exploring thresholds for action in safeguarding.

Michaels, J (2008) *Healthcare for All: Report of the independent inquiry into access to healthcare for people with learning disabilities*. Available online at www.dh.gov.uk/prod_consum_dh/groups/dh_digitalassets/@dh/@en/documents/digitalasset/dh_106126.pdf.

This report highlights the problems that people with learning disabilities face in accessing appropriate healthcare. Many of the recommendations made for this client group can equally apply to other vulnerable people.

O'Keeffe, M, Hills, A, Doyle, M, McCreadie, C, Scholes, S, Constantine, R, Tinker, A, Manthorpe, J, Biggs, S and Erens, B (2007) *UK Study of Abuse and Neglect of Older People: Prevalence survey report*. London: National Centre for Social Research. Available online at http://assets.comicrelief.com/cr09/docs/elderabuseprev.pdf.

This research explores the prevalence of abuse of older people in the UK.

Useful websites

www.pasauk.org.uk/home

Practitioner Alliance for Safeguarding Adults (PASA UK) works in partnership with others engaged in the protection of vulnerable adults and views its work as complementary to that of other statutory and voluntary bodies.

www.respond.org.uk

Respond is an organisation that helps and supports people with learning disabilities who have been abused.

www.voiceuk.org.uk

Voice UK is a national charity that supports vulnerable people who have experienced abuse or crime.

Chapter 5
Safeguarding

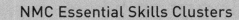

NMC Essential Skills Clusters

This chapter will address the following ESCs:

Cluster: Organisational aspects of care

11. People can trust the newly registered graduate nurse to safeguard children and adults from vulnerable situations and support and protect them from harm.

17. People can trust the newly registered graduate nurse to work safely under pressure and maintain the safety of service users at all times.

18. People can trust a newly registered graduate nurse to enhance the safety of service users and identify and actively manage risk and uncertainty in relation to people, the environment, self and others.

19. People can trust the newly registered graduate nurse to work to prevent and resolve conflict and maintain a safe environment.

Chapter aims

After reading this chapter, you will be able to:

• discuss a 'protection of vulnerable adults' approach to policy and practice;
• explain how a 'safeguarding' approach differs from the 'protection of vulnerable adults';
• identify the key components of a safeguarding approach;
• discuss the implications of safeguarding for the delivery of nursing practice.

Introduction

The number of competencies and essential skills linked to this chapter (see above) should give you an indication of how important safeguarding is to the delivery of professional nursing care: it is a responsibility of every nurse. This chapter will, therefore, introduce you to the concept of safeguarding, and explore its implications for nursing practice. Before you read on, however, take time to complete Activity 5.1 and keep your answer to this activity to hand as you read through the rest of the chapter.

Activity 5.1   *Reflection*

Think about a healthcare setting with which you are familiar and imagine that you are a patient/client using that service.

- What would you want to see put in place to ensure your safety and well-being in that setting?
- What would need to happen for your rights to be upheld?

Try to think about policies, practices and the environment of care.

Some ideas are given at the end of the chapter.

The protection of vulnerable adults

Within the UK we have a relatively long history of having a legal framework to protect children from abuse and neglect. However, it was not until 2000 that England and Wales developed a framework of policy guidance designed to protect adults from abuse. Even then, what was published was 'policy guidance' rather than a clear legal framework, which meant that the guidance was open to local interpretation and implementation (see Chapter 6 for further discussion). Inevitably, policy interpretation and guidance has varied and this has an impact on the extent to which people are protected from abuse or, where abuse occurs, an appropriate, effective and timely response is forthcoming; it is implementation of policy that protects people (Northway et al., 2007). The Commission for Social Care Inspection (2008) examined how effective adult protection policies had been within England. It found uneven progress in the development of effective services, variability in the quality of support provided and variability in terms of action to prevent abuse and achieve better outcomes. The presence of strong leadership, development of strategic partnerships, and a correlation between councils who were performing well and the quality of the care provision within regulated services, were also observed.

The recent consultation document concerning the Social Services (Wales) Bill 2012 thus recognises concerns that adult protection has not had the same attention as child protection, where there is a 'very well-developed and understood legal framework' (Welsh Government, 2012). Relevant legislation will be discussed in Chapter 6, but here we need to consider the term 'protection of vulnerable adults', and how this has developed to the more recent terminology of 'safeguarding'. First take a few minutes to complete Activity 5.2.

Think about the phrase 'protection of vulnerable adults'.

- What does the word 'protection' suggest to you?
- What do you think vulnerable adults might need 'protecting' from?
- How would you feel if you were considered to be a 'vulnerable adult' who was in need of 'protection'?

An outline answer is given at the end of the chapter.

Chapter 2 examined different meanings and understandings of vulnerability. These include it being viewed as a characteristic of an individual, and the idea that individuals may be vulnerable to harm from a range of internal and external factors. In the context of the policy guidance, individuals had to meet the specified criteria, that is, to have certain personal characteristics and to be in receipt of community care services (DH, 2000a; NAfW, 2000). The definition of vulnerable adults as set out in this guidance was, however, challenged on the grounds that it appeared to exclude those who may be vulnerable even though they do not receive community care services (House of Commons Health Committee, 2007).

The term 'vulnerable adult' has become commonly used within health and social care services. It has different meanings in policy guidance, **common law** and **statutes** (Magill et al., 2010). Also, those who are referred to in this manner are not always happy with the terminology (Magill et al., 2010). Support for change was also found in the review of *No Secrets* (DH, 2009b), where 90 per cent of respondents were in favour of changing the definition, and many preferred adoption of the term 'adult at risk' rather than 'vulnerable adult'. In Scotland the Adult Support and Protection (Scotland) Act 2007 does refer to adults 'at risk of harm', and currently within Wales proposals to move to use of similar terminology are being consulted upon (Welsh Government, 2012). Within the Welsh proposals people would be deemed to be at risk if they belong to particular groups (such as people with mental health problems, older people and people with learning disabilities) *and* they are the victim (or potentially the victim) of one or more of the identified forms of harm or abuse. It can been seen that this moves away from the idea that simply by being identified as belonging to a particular group you are inevitably vulnerable: actual or potential harm must also be present.

Safeguarding

The previous section noted that, in relation to children, a legal and policy framework was established in the UK long before any developments took place relating to adults. In terms of supporting children a change in terminology took place and 'child protection' was largely replaced with 'safeguarding'. A similar change has taken place in relation to adults, although the rationale for change may have had a slightly different emphasis. Before exploring this change further take some time to work through Activity 5.3. As you do this try to think of arguments both for and against the issues you identify.

Activity 5.3	*Critical thinking*

- Why do you feel the UK has had a relatively long history of putting measures in place to prevent and respond to the abuse of children, but has only recently started to develop similar measures to protect adults at risk of harm?
- Do you feel it is appropriate to change the terminology to 'safeguarding' in relation to adults as has been the case concerning children?

An outline answer is given at the end of the chapter.

Sometimes a change in terminology is just that: the words change but practice does not. In this context the change is, in part, a response to criticisms that the phrase 'protection of vulnerable adults' was perceived as negative, and as portraying adults as being passive. In addition, policy guidance was often interpreted as addressing abuse and neglect once it has occurred, rather than preventing it from occurring in the first place. In 2005 the Association of Directors of Social Services (ADSS) indicated that the previous terminology would be replaced by 'safeguarding' and this meant:

> all work which enables an adult 'who is or may be eligible for community care services' to retain independence, wellbeing and choice, **and** to access their human right to live a life that is free from abuse and neglect.
> (ADSS, 2005, p5)

The NHS has also adopted the terminology of 'safeguarding', arguing that it is concerned with promoting the safety and well-being of all patients while recognising that those least able to protect themselves from harm may require additional support (DH, 2011a). The Department of Health (2011a) also identifies that safeguarding encompasses a wide range of activities, ranging from prevention of harm and abuse to multi-agency responses when abuse and harm occur. It can thus be seen that it is a rights-based approach that is both proactive and reactive.

Another definition of safeguarding has been proposed by the British Medical Association (BMA):

> Safeguarding is about keeping vulnerable adults safe from harm. It involves identifying adults who may be vulnerable, assessing their needs and working with them and with other agencies in order to protect them from avoidable harms.
> (2011, p11)

Some might criticise this definition for continuing to refer to 'vulnerable adults', but it does introduce two important elements. First, it stresses that safeguarding involves working *with* people who may be vulnerable to harm; it is not about them taking a passive role while others do something to them. Second, it draws attention to the need to be proactive by noting that, in some instances, it is possible to identify the risk of harm and to intervene to prevent it from occurring.

The breadth of the activities involved in safeguarding, and the range of agencies and people who may be involved, are highlighted by the Northern Ireland Office and the Department of Health, Social Services and Public Safety (DHSSPS) (2010). They suggest that, while health, social care and criminal justice agencies have a leading role to play, the involvement of other organisations and agencies across statutory, voluntary, community, private and faith sectors is also required. Safer communities, public transport policies, public health, education and adult learning opportunities are also identified as important elements of successful safeguarding, along with the input of families, carers and good neighbours. It is not the responsibility of one or two statutory agencies – every citizen has a role to play.

Case study: Josh Walsh

Josh is 20 years old and is in his second year at university. During the summer holidays at the end of his first year, his best friend at home was killed in a motorcycle accident. At the time, Josh seemed to be coping reasonably well and went back to university as usual in October. Within a few weeks, however, it became obvious that he was having difficulties. He didn't want to worry his family, who were 150 miles away, and he didn't want to worry his friends at university so he kept things to himself. His results had been good all through his first year but they started to dip, and then he started not handing in work. No matter how hard he tried he just couldn't concentrate, he wasn't eating and he wasn't sleeping; most of his time was spent alone in his room. When he did see other people he tried to behave as though everything was all right; no one noticed that things were wrong. One day another student noticed that he hadn't seen Josh for a few days. He knocked on his door, but there was no answer, so he fetched a member of staff who went with him into Josh's room where they found him in bed, unable to communicate with them. After assessment by the GP Josh was diagnosed as suffering from severe depression, and was admitted to a local mental health unit; he has been there for four weeks. Initially he was withdrawn, but when his mood started to lift he began to express ideas of self-harm and had to be monitored very closely. This now appears to have passed and discussions are taking place in preparation for his discharge. Josh is adamant that he wants to return to university and to get things back to normal.

Activity 5.4   *Critical thinking*

Think about the situation of Josh in the case study above.

- What do you feel needs to be in place to safeguard him from harm when he is discharged?

An outline answer is given at the end of the chapter.

Another important element of safeguarding identified by the Department of Health (2011a) is that of learning from practice, and using this learning to inform future interventions (see Figure 5.1). This is essential in the context of seeking to protect people who may be at risk of harm, since harm will not always be prevented and it is essential that we learn from these situations in order to try to prevent similar situations from occurring in the future. Unfortunately, however, as was seen in Chapter 1, we do not always seem to learn the lessons from inquiries into abuse and poor standards of care, even though the reports of such inquiries note similar findings.

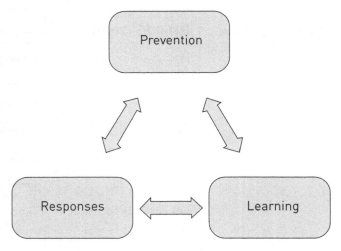

Figure 5.1 Key elements of safeguarding identified by the Department of Health (2011a)

To relate this to your personal practice, take a few minutes to complete Activity 5.5.

Activity 5.5   *Reflection*

Think about a care situation in which you have been involved where a patient or client has come to some harm.

- How was the situation managed?
- What did you learn from the situation?
- Did you learn anything that you could use in your practice to try to prevent a similar situation from occurring in the future?

Some guidance is included at the end of the chapter, but try to address the questions yourself first.

The principles of safeguarding

Most discussions concerning safeguarding make reference to principles or values that underpin the approach and some examples of these are set out in Table 5.1. Looking at the table you will see some principles that were discussed in Chapter 3, where we explored ethical issues; the relationship between ethics and safeguarding should be clear. In Table 5.1 it can be seen that some principles appear in more than one list, for example empowerment and rights. Others are clearly linked, such as justice and legal protection. Some are self-explanatory but others perhaps require some further discussion.

Some of these principles, such as legal protection and rights, will be explored later in this book (see Chapter 6) and the relevance of key legislation to safeguarding will also be discussed there. Other principles will be discussed here before considering their implications for care planning and delivery.

Department of Health (2011a)	DHSSPS (2006)	Reece (2010)
Empowerment	Privacy	Protection
Protection	Respect and dignity	Promotion of well-being
Prevention	Choice	Empowerment
Proportionality	Legal protection	Rights
Partnerships	Rights upheld	Justice
Accountability	Opportunity to realise potential	

Table 5.1 Principles underpinning safeguarding

Protection and the promotion of well-being

Having previously identified that the word 'protection' can be problematic, it also needs to be acknowledged that there are clearly situations where some adults are at risk of harm or abuse. In such circumstances they may need protection from others, themselves or particular situations, and therefore it needs to be included as a principle that informs safeguarding. However, placing protection alongside other important elements recognises that it is an essential part of the overall approach, but that other elements are also required. Protection suggests that a preventative approach is required, as well as a response where abuse has occurred, so as to prevent further harm. The inclusion of 'promotion of well-being' also suggests a wider-ranging approach. Rather than just preventing harm it requires that a positive approach to enhancing well-being is taken. If you refer back to Chapter 3 it can be seen that beneficence and not just non-maleficence is required.

Empowerment

Within healthcare situations patients can often be (or feel they are) less powerful than the health professionals who are working with them. Professionals may be seen as knowledgeable experts and patients are expected to take on a passive role in complying with the professional advice given to them. We have all probably heard people with whom we are working say 'whatever you think is best'. However, this situation makes people vulnerable to loss of control over their own lives, over decisions that are made, and sometimes subject to treatment that they find abusive or harmful. Clearly, there are some situations where people lack the capacity to take control or to express their views and wishes. In such circumstances legal safeguards are required and these will be discussed in Chapter 6. At other times it is important to safeguard against the potential for a lack of control and power by working in an empowering way; empowerment is a key principle underpinning a safeguarding approach.

Empowerment has been defined in a number of ways, but one helpful definition in this context is that provided by Slettebo (2006), who suggests that it is *a process of equipping a person to be in charge of his or her own life* (p115). This shows how it is a developmental process that seeks to increase people's capacity to take control and this in turn gives rise to two points that are important in relation to safeguarding. First, it suggests that, where people appear to be at risk of harm, we can support them to increase their personal capacity and hopefully reduce the risk of harm occurring: their current abilities can be enhanced. Second, where abuse or harm has occurred an empowering approach can be used to reduce feelings of powerlessness that can arise from abuse and also assist people to feel better able to anticipate and manage future risks.

Accountability

It is important to note that the Department of Health (2011a) identifies the need for accountability in relation to safeguarding. Outcome 7 of the Care Quality Commission standards relates specifically to safeguarding from abuse those people who use care services. It states that *People should be protected from abuse, or the risk of abuse, and their human rights are respected and upheld* (CQC, 2010, p93). Unfortunately, however, major concerns have been expressed regarding non-achievement of this standard in some services for people with learning disabilities (CQC, 2012) and moderate concerns have also been identified in acute hospital settings (see the CQC website for up-to-date information at www.cqc.org.uk). Some of the issues to emerge in these reports were a lack of staff training regarding safeguarding, patients feeling at risk from other patients, and a failure to protect patients. Establishments assessed as failing to achieve the necessary standards are given a specified period to respond and to say how they intend to improve the situation.

Proportionality

In some circumstances where harm occurs it is reasonably clear as to what the response should be. For example, if a law has been broken prosecution may be necessary, and if guilt is proven an appropriate sentence is handed down based on official guidelines for the specific offence. However, in other circumstances the required response may be less clear and it is important to know whether to respond, how to respond and what sanctions should be applied. Think about a situation in which a family member comes into a ward and takes £20 of her elderly mother's money without her knowledge or consent. Then think about another situation in which you observe that an elderly lady you have been visiting in the community seems to have little food in the house, her house is cold and she seems to have a lot of unpaid bills. When you discuss this with her you eventually find out that a neighbour who comes to visit her has been collecting your patient's pension, saying that she would pay the bills and get the shopping and take a little bit of money to pay her for her time. Your patient says that she knows this means she doesn't have any money, but she is worried that, without her neighbour helping her, she wouldn't be able to cope. Both of these situations could constitute financial abuse, but should they be dealt with in the same way?

The Department of Health (2011a) identifies 'proportionality' as a key principle underpinning safeguarding, arguing that responses to abuse and harm should be in keeping with the nature and seriousness of the concern. It also stresses that responses should be those that place least restriction on the rights of the individual who has been harmed, taking account of factors such as his or her age, culture, wishes, lifestyle and beliefs. Finally, the Department suggests that proportionality also means that concerns must be addressed in the most effective and efficient manner.

Essence of Care benchmarks

Many of these principles can be seen in other policies that inform the provision of healthcare and this highlights how safeguarding is (or should be) an integral part of healthcare provision. For example, great emphasis has been placed on promoting and monitoring the fundamentals or essence of care. In 2010 the Department of Health published *Essence of Care 2010* (DH, 2010b), which sets out standards for and indicators of quality care. A general principle stated throughout the document relates to safeguarding: *robust, integrated systems are in place to identify and respond to abuse, harm and neglect*. Some of the specific areas discussed link directly to the principles underpinning safeguarding set out in Table 5.1, such as 'Benchmarks for Respect and Dignity' and 'Benchmarks for Promoting Health and Well-Being'. Examples of indicators in each of these areas are set out in Table 5.2.

It should be noted that Table 5.2 includes only examples of some of the many outcomes, factors and indicators of best practice identified by the Department of Health (2010b), and you may wish to look at the relevant document and consider some of the other areas addressed. The examples given do, however, demonstrate a few important points. First, it can be seen that in all areas reference is made to 'people' rather than 'patients', 'service users' or other terms that are frequently used within healthcare settings. This careful choice of words reflects the importance of valuing and respecting all people because they are just that, people. Second, if you read the examples of best practice carefully you will see that the emphasis is on supporting people to take as much control as possible over what happens to them and on the importance of creating environments in which this can happen. People are not viewed as being passive recipients of services that are controlled by healthcare professionals. Instead, they are active partners in the process of healthcare planning and delivery.

Each of the principles set out in this section has implications for the delivery of nursing care and these will be discussed further in the next section. Before you read on, however, take some time to complete Activity 5.6.

Activity 5.6   *Leadership and management*

- Imagine you have just been appointed to manage a clinical area or community team. Take one of the principles set out above and identify how you would ensure that it is upheld within the area you are managing.
- How do you feel that it would help to promote the safeguarding of people who might otherwise be at risk of harm, abuse or neglect?

An outline answer is given at the end of the chapter.

Outcome	Factor	Best practice
People experience care that is focused upon respect	Attitudes and behaviour	People and carers feel that they matter all of the time
	Personal boundaries and space	People's personal space is protected by staff
	Privacy, modesty and dignity	People's care ensures their privacy and dignity and protects their modesty
	Privacy – private area	People and carers can access an area that safely provides privacy
People will be supported to make healthier choices for themselves and others	Assessment	People, carers and communities are enabled to identify their health and well-being promotion needs
	Environment	People, carers, communities and agencies influence and create environments that promote people's health and well-being
	Outcomes of promoting health and well-being	People, carers and communities have an improved, sustainable and good-quality health and well-being

Table 5.2 Essence of Care *benchmarks (DH, 2010b)*

Safeguarding in practice

As has already been seen in this chapter there are a number of levels at which different responsibilities for safeguarding can be seen to operate. These are set out in Figure 5.2.

Individual level

As nurses we are all responsible and accountable for our practice, and for ensuring that we are fit for practice. Our *Code* (NMC, 2008a, pp3–7) identifies a number of areas that are related to our safeguarding responsibilities, such as the following.

- You must disclose information if you believe someone may be at risk of harm, in line with the law of the country in which you are practising.
- You must respect and support people's rights to accept or decline treatment and care.
- You must be able to demonstrate that you have acted in someone's best interests if you have provided care in an emergency.
- You must act immediately to put matters right if someone in your care has suffered harm for any reason.
- You must act without delay if you believe that you, a colleague or anyone else may be putting someone at risk.
- You must inform someone in authority if you experience problems that prevent you working within this code or other nationally agreed standards.
- You must report your concerns in writing if problems in the environment of care are putting people at risk.

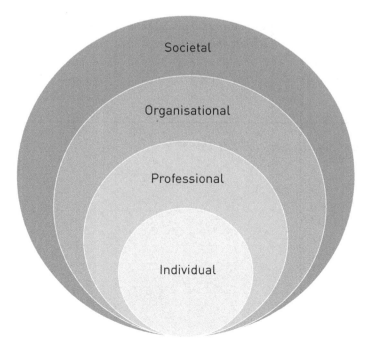

Figure 5.2 Levels of responsibility for safeguarding

However, despite these clear links between our *Code* and our safeguarding responsibilities, it has been suggested that nurses remain unclear as to their responsibilities in relation to safeguarding (Draper et al., 2009; Straughair, 2011). The Department of Health (2011a) has therefore developed guidance that focuses on the role of health service practitioners. Within this document it identifies themes that have recurred in recent 'high-profile' inquiries into failures of care (see Chapter 2).

If such situations are to be prevented we all, as individual practitioners, have responsibilities. For example, we need to accept that we all have a responsibility for safeguarding adults who are in our care or whom we support. Our employers, other agencies and other professionals do have a role, but this does not excuse us from accepting responsibility for our own contribution. If we are to work in empowering ways we need to enable patients and clients to exercise as much control over their lives as possible, recognising that, at times, their health status may limit the extent to which this is possible and that, at times, there may be legal restrictions (see Chapter 6). At a practical level this might include making sure that they have access to accurate and timely information made available in a format, and at a pace, that enables them to understand. Using simple, clear language, providing audio and not just written formats, using Braille, translation into other languages, and using pictures rather than words, may all be required to meet individual information needs. Empowerment might also involve working with patients and clients to develop their confidence in managing their health, to enhance their assertiveness skills or to recognise threats to their health and well-being.

It is important to note that the themes identified by the Department of Health (2011a) include recognition that patients' voices are not always heard. This highlights how an empowering approach to safeguarding requires that we, as individual practitioners, also need to examine (and if necessary change) our behaviour. For example, are there examples of situations where we have taken away someone's power by not really listening to him or her? It may be that the person has been trying to take control over a situation by telling us something he or she feels is important but, while we have heard what the person says, we have not really listened. The person's power has been reduced because we have not really understood what he or she has been trying to tell us and therefore have not acted on it. We also need to remember that people can 'tell' us things in other ways; it is not just what they say. Body language, mood and facial expressions can all be powerful ways of communicating, but we need to be alert to these and seek to understand their significance, thus increasing the control that patients have over what happens to them.

The Department of Health (2011a) suggests that neglect and abuse are not always recognised by healthcare staff. However, if we accept that we all have a responsibility for safeguarding adults, it follows that we need to understand exactly what constitutes abuse and neglect. Also, if inquiries into failures of care highlight a lack of transparency in relation to investigations, it also follows that as individuals we have a duty to ensure that we are aware of our responsibilities for identifying and reporting suspected abuse and neglect in line with agreed procedures. Furthermore, it is important that we make ourselves aware *before* we encounter such incidents as this will increase both our confidence and competence in what can be a difficult situation.

It is also important to recognise that we have a duty in preventing abuse and neglect; we have a proactive as well as a reactive role. The Department of Health (2011a) suggests that there are two main areas we need to consider here. First, we need to work with the patients and clients we are supporting to help them recognise and reduce risks to their health and well-being. This might include working with patients and their families to understand how they perceive risk. It also requires that both the benefits and the possible disadvantages of taking risks are considered (DH, 2011a). The second area we need to focus on is preventing neglect, harm and abuse within healthcare settings (DH, 2011a). This requires that, at all times, we treat individuals with dignity and respect and that we are prepared to challenge and report poor practice if we observe it or its effects.

Professional level

The nursing profession within the UK is regulated by the Nursing and Midwifery Council (NMC). The key aim of this organisation is *to safeguard the health and well-being of the public* (NMC, 2010a). This is achieved via a range of activities, including setting and monitoring standards of professional education, maintaining the professional register, setting professional standards for practice and providing guidance, and investigating and hearing cases of professional misconduct. Each of these areas has significance in relation to safeguarding.

In setting the standards for professional education, the NMC (2010c) has outlined explicit standards relating to safeguarding and others that have relevance to safeguarding, as can be seen at the beginning of each of the chapters in this book. All universities providing nursing education thus have to ensure that the curriculum they deliver includes appropriate theoretical and practical experience to ensure that students are able to meet the required standards in these and other areas.

All registered nurses are required to renew their registration every three years and, in doing so, they are required not only to pay a registration fee but also to declare that they have undergone required periods of professional updating. This register can be checked online, meaning that employers and even members of the public are able to check the registration status of individual practitioners.

The *Code* (NMC, 2008a) sets out the key standards against which nursing practice is assessed and identifies the responsibilities of all nurses. Some of these relate specifically to safeguarding, while others relate to other areas of nursing practice. Some identify how a nurse's personal practice must be safe, competent and delivered in a professional manner so as to protect the health and well-being of patients and clients. However, it is also stressed that, where the environment of care means that nurses cannot practise in this manner, they must inform relevant persons in authority and put their concerns in writing. Also, if they or another person places a person at risk, they should then act without delay. Although a professional requirement, raising such concerns can be very difficult and the NMC has subsequently issued further guidance on *Raising and Escalating Concerns* (NMC, 2010b). Within this document it is stressed that practitioners raising a genuine concern will be viewed as upholding professional responsibilities. A failure to report concerns is 'unacceptable': such a failure to act could bring into question the nurse's continued fitness to practise and place his or her registration at risk.

Where professional misconduct is suspected, nurses are reported to the NMC, which has a duty to investigate and to hold a hearing. Outcomes of such hearings can include the nurse being removed or suspended from the register.

Organisational level

Although safeguarding has now become a more widely integrated part of NHS provision, it has been suggested that as an organisation the NHS has demonstrated a lack of ownership of safeguarding (DH et al., 2009). Some of the healthcare organisations responding to the consultation concerning a review of *No Secrets* indicated that there was a widely held perception that care provided by health professionals is 'safe', although the report also cites examples indicating that this is not always the case (DH et al., 2009). The Department of Health (2011a) subsequently notes that individual practitioners cannot effectively manage concerns relating to safeguarding adults without the support of their service. It is important that healthcare organisations develop and maintain systems, structures and a culture in which safeguarding is recognised as a central concern. Some of these features will be explored in more detail in Chapters 8 and 9. In this chapter we do, however, need to look at some of these issues.

Healthcare organisations are often large and complex, employing many staff. While we are concerned here primarily with nurses, it is important to remember that *all* staff have responsibilities in relation to safeguarding. It is therefore important that organisations do all they can to make sure that the staff they recruit have the personal and professional characteristics required. This involves ensuring that references are taken up and that checks are made to confirm that references are genuine. Pre-employment checks in relation to criminal records need to be undertaken. Where professional registration is a requirement of a post, checks need to be made to ensure that such registration is current and has not lapsed. Interview procedures need to be carefully structured so as to make certain that key requirements of the post are tested while observing the demands of relevant legislation (for example, relating to equalities).

Clearly, duties relating to employees do not end once someone is in post, and organisations need to ensure that appropriate training is provided relating to safeguarding responsibilities and that such training is provided on a regular basis. This training needs to include issues such as the nature of abuse and neglect, the principles of safeguarding, and individual responsibilities in relation to responding to and reporting abuse. Clear policies and standards need to be in place and monitoring of such standards needs to occur. Where poor practice does occur, mechanisms need to be in place to ensure that it does not recur (Morgan, 2010).

Should harm, neglect or abuse take place, it is essential that lessons are learnt so that potential areas for change can be identified, thus reducing future risks. Clinical supervision can be one way of facilitating reflection on such incidents (Morgan, 2010) and this can be a helpful basis for both individual and organisational learning. Organisations therefore need to ensure that clinical supervision is an integral part of their staff support systems.

As noted above, organisations need to have policies in place that clearly set out the steps to be taken should harm, abuse or neglect be suspected. Each area will have its own such policy and it is essential that you take time to acquaint yourself with this policy and to seek clarification if any aspects are unclear. However, in setting out the broad responsibilities of organisations, the Department of Health (2011a) advocates a 'stepped' approach. Such an approach and its practice implications are set out in Figure 5.3.

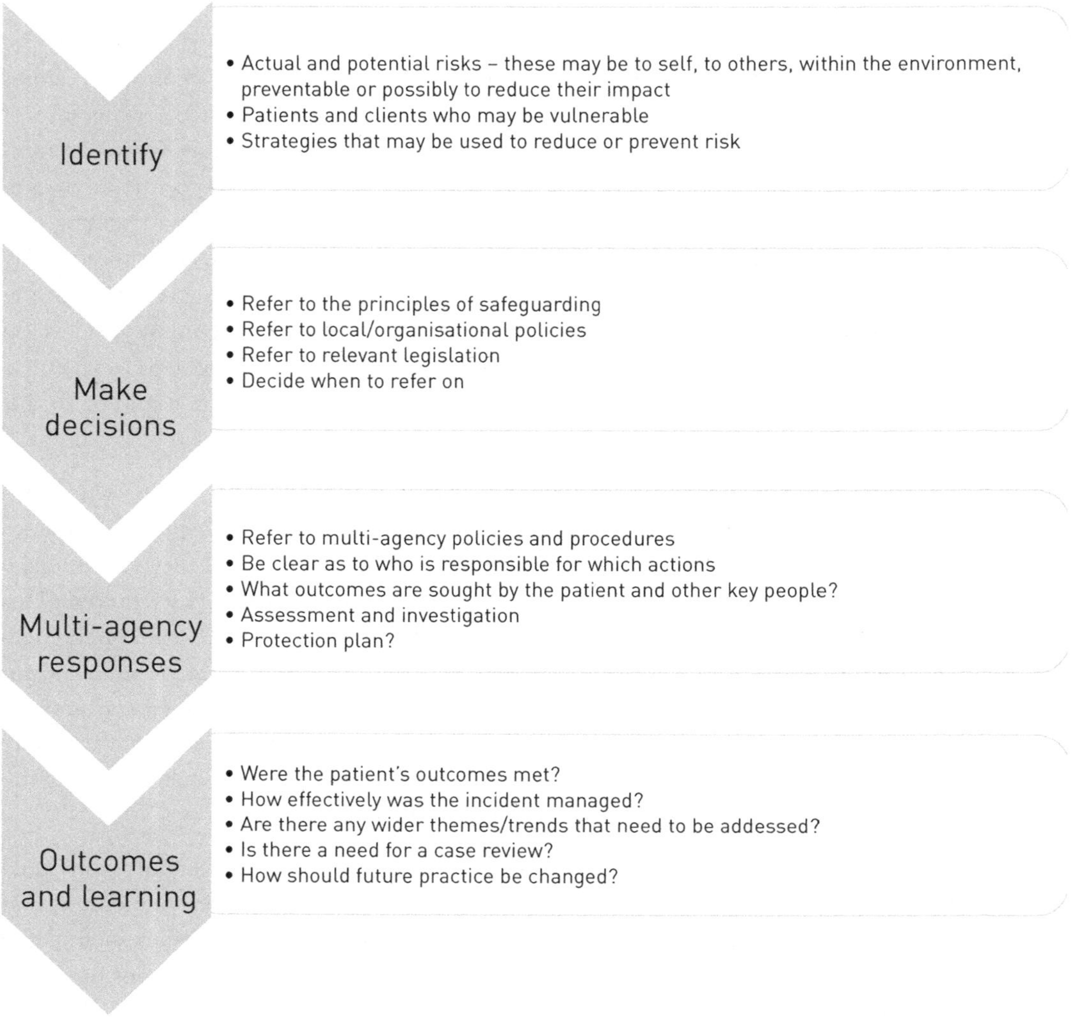

Identify
- Actual and potential risks – these may be to self, to others, within the environment, preventable or possibly to reduce their impact
- Patients and clients who may be vulnerable
- Strategies that may be used to reduce or prevent risk

Make decisions
- Refer to the principles of safeguarding
- Refer to local/organisational policies
- Refer to relevant legislation
- Decide when to refer on

Multi-agency responses
- Refer to multi-agency policies and procedures
- Be clear as to who is responsible for which actions
- What outcomes are sought by the patient and other key people?
- Assessment and investigation
- Protection plan?

Outcomes and learning
- Were the patient's outcomes met?
- How effectively was the incident managed?
- Are there any wider themes/trends that need to be addessed?
- Is there a need for a case review?
- How should future practice be changed?

Figure 5.3 A stepped approach to safeguarding (adapted from DH, 2011a)

It can be seen in Figure 5.3 that individual, professional and organisational responsibilities all come together in a stepped approach to safeguarding. To apply this to practice, take some time to read through the case study of Emily Saunders and then complete Activity 5.7.

Case study: Emily Saunders

Emily is 25 years old and lives with two other people of a similar age. She likes loud music, enjoys going to the cinema and loves ice cream. She has an infectious laugh and often finds things funny. Emily has severe learning and physical disabilities; she cannot communicate verbally and needs to use a wheelchair if she goes out. She also has epilepsy. As she and her housemates need assistance with most aspects of daily living, there are usually two staff supporting them at all times.

continued . . .

*Yesterday Emily came into the hospital's A&E department supported by a member of staff. Her support staff had noticed that she had been very withdrawn and irritable, that she seemed to be experiencing some abdominal pain, and that she had some blood in her stools. When she arrived at A&E the staff member who came with her said that she would need to return to the house as she had left the other member of staff alone. She gave the nurse Emily's **hospital passport** and said that this document would provide the staff with the information they needed to look after Emily. She apologised, however, that Emily's medication had recently been changed and that the passport had not been updated to reflect this. She wrote the name of the new medication on a piece of paper and said that it was important to give Emily her tablets in the right order – the big tablet first and then the small tablet. Having been assessed in A&E, it was decided that Emily should be admitted for observation and investigations. When she was transferred to the ward the staff were informed of Emily's hospital passport and the admitting nurse read it before slipping it into the case file. It was her intention to use the information in the passport to develop Emily's care plan, but as she was going off duty a colleague said that she would do the care plan. Unfortunately, the first nurse forgot to tell her colleague about the hospital passport and so this information was not used to develop a plan that reflected her needs. At teatime a meal was put in front of Emily, but the staff did not initially realise that she needed assistance with eating. When they finally went to assist her the food was cold; also, it was cottage pie and carrots: Emily hates carrots and pushed the staff and the food away. Information about her support needs and likes and dislikes was in her hospital passport. She was not offered any drink and the nurse who assisted her thought it wouldn't be a problem as someone else would help her to have a drink later. This didn't happen. When she was given her medication she refused to take it as the tablets were given together in a medication cup.*

During the evening Emily became very distressed and the staff tried without success to calm her. In fact, Emily needed to go to the toilet and her shouting had been her usual way of telling other people about her need. When she was incontinent she became even more distressed, particularly when the nurse told her she should have asked to go to the toilet. Also, she was in pain and she was trying to tell the staff this by rocking and screaming. Again, this information was in the hospital passport. Overnight Emily became increasingly more distressed; the nursing staff believed that this was due to her learning disability. In the morning the nurse in charge telephoned the house staff to say that Emily was being discharged as they had been unable to find a cause for her current problems. The support staff have arrived on the ward to find Emily in an extremely agitated and distressed state and they are still concerned that she is unwell.

Activity 5.7   *Communication and decision making*

Read through Emily Saunders' case study.

- Were Emily's health and well-being safeguarded?
- How did breakdowns in communication contribute to a breakdown in care?
- To what extent did poor communication lead to poor decision making?
- Go through the various stages in this case study and suggest ways in which communication could have been improved and more effective care could have been provided.

Some discussion is included at the end of the chapter to assist you.

Societal level

Harm, abuse and neglect occur within the context of society and, while individuals, professionals and organisations such as the health service have responsibilities in relation to safeguarding adults, communities and wider society also have a key role to play. For example, the Department of Health (2011b) suggests a focus on community empowerment and localism. This involves communities making decisions as to what their priorities are, including how adults at risk of harm may best be protected. The Northern Ireland Office and the Department of Health, Social Services and Public Safety (DHSSPS, 2010) also see an important role for local communities, noting that all citizens have a responsibility to safeguard vulnerable adults through being aware of danger signs, and also acting on their concerns should they suspect abuse or neglect. They view a range of community-based agencies such as housing, public transport and adult education as having a key role to play, as well as members of the public supporting individuals and families through acts of good neighbourliness and citizenship.

For the wider public to be aware of their potential role in relation to safeguarding requires, however, that they are provided with information concerning both the nature of abuse and neglect, and the potential role they can play. The health service and healthcare practitioners, including nurses, have a key role to play in raising general awareness about neglect and abuse along with providing information about how to raise concerns.

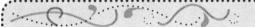

Chapter summary

This chapter has examined the protection of vulnerable adults and the reasons for moving towards a safeguarding approach. The broader nature of safeguarding has been explored, stressing that it encompasses both a proactive and reactive approach to harm, abuse and neglect. The principles that underpin safeguarding have been examined and some implications of a safeguarding approach for the development of practice considered. A 'stepped' approach is advocated with action required at individual, professional, organisational and societal levels. Responsibilities at each of these levels and the interaction between the levels have been explored.

Activities: Brief outline answers

Activity 5.1 Reflection, page 87

Your answer to this activity will inevitably depend on the particular area you decided to focus on and your particular needs. However, following are some of the things you might have identified.

- **Policies** – You might want to know that there are agreed policies in place for things such as seeking consent, dealing with confidential information, reporting any adverse incidents, checking the professional status of staff, and record keeping.
- **Practices** – You might want assurance that staff are competent to carry out the interventions required; you might want to know that the care you receive is considered 'best practice'; and you might expect your care to be carried out in a way that protects your dignity, is respectful and recognises your individuality.

- **The environment of care** – You might want to ensure that any equipment used is safe, that you can be afforded privacy, that you are not subjected to undue noise, that there is good communication, that your nutritional and hydration needs will be met, that infection risks are minimised and that you are not at risk of harm.

Activity 5.2 Critical thinking, page 88

In Chapter 2 we examined some different ways of understanding 'vulnerability' and it was seen that, while some may view vulnerability as an inevitable part of belonging to certain groups, others view it as something that can be prevented or minimised. In this context, however, the phrase 'protection of vulnerable adults' has been criticised for portraying a passive view of those to whom the label is applied. Being in need of protection can be viewed as a weakness and it can be stigmatising. While we may use this terminology to refer to people we support, we might perhaps feel uncomfortable at the thought of the label being applied to us. It is important to recognise this and to increase our understanding of why some people we support find it difficult to accept some of the labels that are applied to them by services.

Activity 5.3 Critical thinking, page 89

Concerns are often expressed about drawing too many parallels between addressing abuse, harm and neglect that occurs to adults and that which occurs to children. Legally, there are differences (see Chapter 6) but also it is generally felt important to recognise that adults (generally) have greater autonomy and that they are often better able to protect themselves from harm. Nonetheless, the term 'safeguarding' describes an approach that is broader than just responding to abuse, neglect and harm when it occurs: a proactive approach is also included with an emphasis on prevention. Safeguarding has therefore gained wider acceptance in relation to supporting adults at risk of harm, since it is felt to be less stigmatising and it includes prevention.

Activity 5.4 Critical thinking, page 90

It is important to undertake an assessment of Josh's current mental health state and his risk of self-harm. Before his discharge from hospital it will also be important to work with Josh to ensure that a plan is in place to provide support. This may include the support of community nurses, psychologists or regular contact with therapeutic services such as counselling. It will also be important to work with him to identify any triggers for his recent illness and any signs that, with hindsight, were an indication that things were wrong. This information can then be used to try to avoid triggers or manage them more effectively, and the signs can be documented in a relapse plan that Josh (and others who support him) can use to recognise if his health is deteriorating again. It will be important to ensure that he has people to support him and that he and his supporters know who to contact if problems arise.

Activity 5.5 Reflection, page 91

Obviously we do not want harm, abuse or neglect to occur, but unfortunately sometimes such incidents do happen. What is important is that we learn from these incidents and use that learning to avoid future problems. When you thought of the incident in this activity, were you aware of a procedure that was followed and any forms that had to be completed? What happened to any forms? Were they looked at to identify learning points and was this information fed back to the clinical area? For example, if an elderly patient with dementia has had a fall as a result of wandering from the ward, can we learn anything about how best to observe patients with dementia? If a disabled patient fails to receive adequate hydration as a consequence of not being able to reach a glass of water, can we learn anything about the positioning of the glass and other equipment and the importance of checking with the patient how he or she would like things placed to best meet his or her needs? If a patient with mental health problems is abused by another patient, what can we learn about better risk assessment and staff support?

Activity 5.6 Leadership and management, page 94

Again, your answer will depend on which principle you decided to focus on. However, if we take empowerment as an example, you might promote this in a clinical setting in a variety of ways, including:

* making sure that information is available for patients and families in formats that are accessible to them;
* taking time to explain things to patients and families;
* not assuming that you know best and instead working in partnership with patients and their families to plan and deliver care;
* supporting patients to remain self-caring wherever possible to avoid loss of skills;
* making sure that patients who need them have access to their glasses, hearing aids and wheelchairs;
* ensuring that new staff are inducted into this approach to care;
* challenging staff if they do not work in an empowering way;
* making sure that patients and families know how to raise concerns about care and that they feel able to do so without fear of it adversely affecting their care.

Activity 5.7 Communication and decision making, page 101

This case study highlights how one breakdown in communication can be compounded by subsequent errors that have a cumulative effect on patient care. Individual mistakes can easily occur and in isolation may not have a major impact. However, when taken together they can have severe effects.

The house staff had been proactive in developing a hospital passport for Emily and this should have assisted the hospital staff, but it had not been updated to reflect recent changes. The staff member was unable to remain with Emily and thus the only source of information the hospital had was the passport. But this was never used and most staff were unaware of its existence. As a result, Emily did not receive care that met her needs and her behaviour deteriorated. This was seen as a consequence of her learning disability, rather than as the result of a failure to understand her ways of communicating her needs and a failure to address her pain. Her needs were neglected and she was sent home without any resolution regarding her health problems.

You might wish to rewrite this case study showing how good communication could lead to a positive outcome for Emily.

Further reading

British Medical Association (BMA) (2011) *Safeguarding Vulnerable Adults: A toolkit for general practitioners.* Available online at www.bma.org.uk/ethics/doctor_relationships/safeguardvulnerableadults.jsp.

This document explores definitions, practice implications and legal issues.

Department of Health (DH) (2011) *Safeguarding Adults: The role of health service practitioners.* Available online at www.dh.gov.uk/publications.

This document expands on many of the points discussed in this chapter.

Pritchard, J (2008) *Good Practice in Safeguarding Adults: Working effectively in adult protection.* London: Jessica Kingsley.

This book is a good overview of adult safeguarding.

Reece, A (2010) Leading the change from adult protection to safeguarding adults: more than just semantics. *Journal of Adult Protection*, 12(3): 30–4.

This paper explores the change in terminology discussed in this chapter.

Useful websites

www.cqc.org.uk

On the Care Quality Commission website you can review the outcomes of the various inspections undertaken. One standard relates specifically to safeguarding.

www.nmc-uk.org

The NMC website provides information regarding professional standards and regulation.

Chapter 6
Legal and policy provisions

continued . . .

v. Is acceptant of differing cultural traditions, beliefs, UK legal frameworks and professional ethics when planning care with people and their families and carers.

7. People can trust a newly qualified graduate nurse to protect and keep as confidential all information relating to them.

By entry to the register:

viii. Works within the legal frameworks for data protection including access to and storage of records.

ix. Acts within the law when confidential information has to be shared with others.

8. People can trust the newly registered graduate nurse to gain their consent based on sound understanding and informed choice prior to any intervention and that their rights in decision making and consent will be respected and upheld.

By entry to the register:

v. Works within legal frameworks when seeking consent.

vii. Demonstrates respect for the autonomy and rights of people to withhold consent in relation to treatment within legal frameworks and in relation to people's safety.

Chapter aims

After reading this chapter, you will be able to:

* discuss the importance of policy and legislation in safeguarding adults at risk of harm and the tension between protection and empowerment;
* identify key provisions of legislation relevant to safeguarding;
* recognise some barriers that may limit the impact of policy and legislation;
* understand the need for nurses to work within legal and policy frameworks.

Introduction

Policy and legislation are important tools in safeguarding people from harm and abuse and, since safeguarding is a role that nurses are required to perform, it is important that they are aware of relevant policy and legislation, and that they recognise situations in which they need to be used. This is what this chapter focuses on.

Remember, however, that the UK comprises four countries and, since devolution, differences in both policy and legislation are increasing between countries, so it is important that you understand the policy and legislation that applies in the country in which you are practising. Also, books are written at a specific point in time, but policy and legislation are in a constant state of development. This means that you always need to check that you are referring to, and working in keeping with, the most recent developments. Some further reading and useful websites are provided at the end of the chapter to help you with this.

The role of policy and legislation

Social policies are a response to social problems or issues that are felt by society to require some form of action. Examples of such issues include healthcare, housing, welfare benefits and, of course, the protection of adults at risk of abuse and neglect. Hill (2009) suggests that *the concept of policy is vague and elusive* (p19), but identifies key features that recur in common definitions, including:

- making reference to a series of decisions that represent a position on a given topic;
- that policy itself develops over time and builds upon previous policies;
- having aims by which 'success' may be determined;
- that non-decision making may be an important element, and it includes both decisions and actions.

The last feature may appear confusing as you probably think of policies as being about 'doing' something. However, sometimes a deliberate decision is made not to take action about a problem, and this decision itself becomes a significant action. It is therefore interesting to think about the areas in which we have policy, and the areas we do not. For example, why have we only had policies relating to the protection of vulnerable adults for a relatively short period of time, compared with law and policy relating to child protection? Has the abuse of adults only occurred for the past 10–15 years, or is it that it is only during this period that it has been recognised as an issue where action is required?

Some see policy development as a very rational, structured process that identifies problems, reviews different solutions and adopts the 'best' option, which is then implemented. Others argue that major changes are not made but, instead, smaller-scale 'incremental' changes are tried and, if they work, further small changes are introduced. Both these approaches are 'ideal' models and in practice things rarely work out in such a manner. Power operates in the policy process where some people or groups have more power than others and are therefore able to exert more influence. Burke et al. (2009) argue that it is a complex and untidy process that does not occur in a rational manner. They further suggest that the decisions involved, which evolve over time (including the implementation process), can be likened to a 'web'.

Earlier chapters of this book have shown how inquiries into failures in care led eventually to recognition of a problem requiring a formal policy response to safeguard adults (DH, 2000a; NAfW, 2000). This development built upon other policy initiatives such as those developed in relation to child protection. While the policy did not prescribe what had to happen, it did set out a framework within which recommended actions should occur.

Within England, Wales and Northern Ireland a policy framework to support the protection of vulnerable adults was introduced rather than specific legislation. In contrast, Scotland introduced legislation that seeks to safeguard adults who are at risk and who are unable to safeguard their own interests (the Adult Support and Protection (Scotland) Act 2007). This legislation places a duty on local authorities to make inquiries where someone is thought to be at risk, including giving them power of entry to premises to make such inquiries. They can also make assessment orders (taking someone elsewhere for the purpose of assessment), removal orders (taking the person out of the setting for up to seven days) and banning orders (banning an alleged perpetrator from the premises and the area) as required. There have been calls for similar legislation in England (DH, 2009b) and Wales (Magill et al., 2010), where proposals for such legislation have been included in the recent Social Services (Wales) Bill consultation document (Welsh Government, 2012). What, then, are the differences between policy and legislation?

Policy sets out a plan or guide as to how services, organisations and procedures should develop. It may, or may not, include provision for monitoring to see whether or not the intended aims have been achieved. Sometimes it is put in place before relevant legislation is developed, but other policies do not develop beyond this level. Most importantly, while policy may set out what is wanted, there are fewer powers to enforce it and implementation often varies.

In contrast, law seeks to regulate behaviour through rules and regulations that can be used to claim rights, create obligations and impose sanctions for non-compliance (Buka, 2008). Griffith and Tengnah (2010) suggest that law comprises a set of rules that are viewed as binding on a given community. These rules may be 'positive' (they impose a legal obligation to either do something or not to do something with sanctions being applied for not obeying such rules) or 'normative' (where they set out what a person should or should not do, but where sanctions are not applied if the desired actions are not taken). They go on to discuss how, within the context of healthcare, both positive and normative rules operate. The law sets out what is required as a minimum standard of care, but as nurses our professional *Code* (NMC, 2008a) requires the highest possible standard of care and it is against this that we are judged. This is an important point to consider when thinking about how best to safeguard those in our care. Take a few minutes to complete Activity 6.1.

Activity 6.1   *Decision making*

Following the exposure of abuse within Winterbourne View Hospital (see Chapter 1, pages 12–13), the Care Quality Commission (2012) undertook a review of learning disability residential services (hospital, assessment units and residential units provided by the NHS, the independent sector and local authorities). It focused its assessment on two of the specified service outcomes, one of which was 'Safeguarding people who use services from abuse'. In relation to this outcome, 79 per cent of NHS settings, 59 per cent of adult social care settings and 51 per cent of independent sector providers were compliant. Major concerns were found in some settings.

Policies regarding safeguarding were in place as were standards against which the services could be assessed. Nonetheless, a significant number of services were failing to meet these standards.

- If you were a nurse working in one of these settings, what would your responsibilities have been?
- What actions should you have taken?

Further discussion regarding this activity is included at the end of the chapter.

In relation to Activity 6.1, it is important to note that policies may not always ensure that intended standards are achieved, and that a failure to achieve standards in relation to safeguarding has significant professional implications for nurses.

There are, broadly, two sources of law in the UK. The first is referred to as 'statutes' and these are laws established by the European Union, the UK Parliament and, increasingly, the devolved administrations of the countries of the UK. The second form of law is referred to as 'case law' or 'common law', and this refers to the decisions made by the courts when they interpret legislation in the context of individual cases. When making decisions, courts consider existing legislation and previous cases tried under the same laws and then arrive at their decision. This decision then forms what is called a 'precedent', which (if it differs from previous decisions in similar cases) in effect develops the law, and this then informs decision making in future cases. It is also important to note that, in some instances, codes of practice are issued following the passing of legislation to provide information as to how the legislation should be implemented. Some examples of such codes will be referred to later in this chapter.

Key legislation

Here some of the key legislation relating to vulnerability, abuse and safeguarding will be discussed, and each of the examples given has implications for nursing practice. Advice regarding further reading is provided at the end of the chapter.

Human Rights Act 1998

If abuse is a violation of people's rights (NAfW, 2000) we need to understand human rights and the role that legislation plays in safeguarding such rights if we are to prevent abuse. The Human Rights Act 1998 is the means by which the European Convention on Human Rights was incorporated into UK law. It places a responsibility on public bodies (such as the NHS) to uphold specified rights and also to protect people from the actions of others that may breach such rights (Mantell, 2008). Some specified rights (for example, article 2 – the right to life) are said to be 'absolute', which means that they must be upheld in all circumstances. Other rights are 'qualified', which means that in some circumstances they can be overridden. An example of this is the right to respect for private and family life (article 8) where, if it is suspected that a vulnerable person is being abused within the family, a local authority would be justified in making inquiries into the family situation.

Take some time to work through Activity 6.2 before reading on.

Activity 6.2   *Critical thinking*

- Think about both your own clinical experience and accounts you have come across of care provided within healthcare settings and think about whether you feel the human rights of patients and clients are ever ignored or denied.
- Can you identify any specific areas of practice where upholding human rights can be challenging?

There is further discussion below and at the end of the chapter.

There are many areas of practice that can potentially impinge upon people's rights and the Department of Health (2008) has identified some examples linked to the Human Rights Act 1998 (Table 6.1).

While these rights are set out in UK legislation, it is important to remember that people can only claim their rights if they know what they are. Without this knowledge they cannot know when their rights have been violated or be aware of the protection that is offered by the law. To think about the implications of this, spend some time working on Activity 6.3.

Article	Possible issues relating to healthcare
Article 2: the right to life	• Do not attempt resuscitation (DNAR) orders • Refusal of life-saving treatment • Active or passive euthanasia • Advance directives • Deaths through negligence
Article 3: prohibition of torture	• Physical and mental abuse • Soiled or unchanged sheets • Leaving trays of food in front of people who are unable to eat independently • Using excessive force to restrain patients • Staff not being protected from violence and abuse
Article 8: respect for private and family life	• Privacy on wards • Family visits • Personal and sexual relationships • Personal records • Separation of families due to residential care placements

Table 6.1 The Human Rights Act 1998 and healthcare (DH, 2008)

Activity 6.3   *Reflection*

- Ask your family and friends if they can identify what rights they have under the Human Rights Act 1998.
- Having done this, try to think about whether the patients and clients you work with are likely to know what rights they have under this Act.

Further discussion is included below and at the end of the chapter.

When you undertook Activity 6.3, it is unlikely that your family and friends were able to name their rights (unless, of course, they are lawyers!). This means that many patients, clients and carers with whom you come into contact may also lack awareness. Nurses, therefore, need to ensure both that they are aware of human rights and that they actively seek to promote and safeguard them. Even if people are aware of their legal rights, they may not have the financial or other resources to pursue a case to uphold these rights. In such instances it is important that nurses are aware of potential sources of specialist support for such patients and clients. The important role of the nurse as an advocate can clearly be seen here.

Mental Capacity Act 2005

The Mental Capacity Act 2005 applies to England and Wales. In Scotland there is similar legislation called the Adults with Incapacity (Scotland) Act 2000. Northern Ireland is currently in the process of developing legislation in relation to mental capacity. Within the Mental Capacity Act 2005 there are a number of key provisions that have implications for safeguarding, and four key areas will be examined here – capacity and consent; advance decisions to refuse treatment; deprivation of liberty; and ill-treatment and wilful neglect. The Mental Capacity Act 2005 is also an example of legislation where there is an accompanying *Code of Practice* (Department of Constitutional Affairs, 2007).

Case study: Luke Absalom

Luke is 18 years old, is profoundly deaf and communicates by means of sign language, although he is able to lip read. He has been knocked off his bike and has damaged both his arms. He has been brought into hospital via ambulance but the paramedics say that they 'can't get anything out of him', suggesting that either he is in shock or he has some kind of 'mental problem'. When the staff start to assess Luke he becomes quite agitated. He can understand some of what they say by lip reading, but not everyone is looking at him as they speak. He then sees someone coming towards him with a syringe and gets even more agitated as he has an allergy to penicillin but has no way of telling them. Staff interpret this as aggression and further evidence that he has a 'mental problem'. They suggest that he is not able to consent to treatment, and that he should be sedated so that they can treat him. Finally, someone looks in the pocket of his jacket and finds a card saying that he is deaf and that he can lip read if people look directly at him. Using this approach, and getting him to nod for yes and shake his head for no, they establish why he doesn't want the injection and an alternative is provided.

Activity 6.4   *Communication*

Think about the case study above.

- What were some of the assumptions held by the staff about Luke's behaviour?
- What effect did this have on his care?
- What might have been the outcome if they had not found the card?

Further discussion is included below and at the end of the chapter.

In completing Activity 6.4, it is important to note the need to consider a range of factors when seeking consent to treatment. The next section discusses the provisions within the Mental Capacity Act 2005 relating to this.

Capacity and consent

Historically, assumptions have been made about the capacity of some groups of people to give consent to treatment. Such groups include people with learning disabilities, people with mental health problems, people with dementia and older people. These assumptions have led to two situations, both of which might be viewed as abusive. First, it has sometimes been assumed that no one within these groups would be capable of giving consent and therefore it was acceptable just to provide treatment without the consent of the individual. Sometimes family members or carers would be asked to give consent (although legally one adult cannot give consent for another). The other situation is one where it is assumed that no one within these groups is able to give consent and therefore cannot be treated. As a consequence, people have been left untreated, suffering pain and discomfort.

The starting point for the Mental Capacity Act 2005 is that capacity should be presumed unless there is reason to suspect this is not the case. It also recognises that, while people may not be able to make an informed decision about one thing, they may be able to make an informed decision about something else. For example, a person with dementia may not be able to make an informed decision about taking a new medication, but may be able to decide about whether they wish to go out for a walk. If it is suspected that someone does not have the capacity to make a specific decision, an assessment is required to determine if he or she can:

- understand the information provided;
- retain this information;
- use or weigh up this information to make a decision;
- communicate his or her decision in some way.

If the person can satisfy these criteria, he or she is viewed as having capacity to make that decision even if the decision made is viewed as unwise by others.

In assessing these criteria, however, it is important that efforts are made to present information in a manner that is as accessible as possible to the individual and that different means of communicating his or her wishes have been noted. For example, some people with complex physical disorders may communicate by facial expressions or by eye blinking rather than via the spoken or written word. If, having taken steps to accommodate differing communication approaches, a person cannot meet these criteria, it can be concluded that for this specific decision he or she lacks capacity. Should this be the case, 'best interest' decisions may need to be taken. Where possible, this process should take account of what is known about the views and preferences of the individual. It must not be motivated by a desire to hasten death, and should include relevant people such as the healthcare team, the individual's family or other carers who know the person well. Where there are no family members, an **Independent Mental Capacity Advocate** (IMCA) may be appointed to represent the interests of the individual. The aim is to take a decision in what is felt to be the best interests of the individual.

Advance decisions to refuse treatment

Some people have very strong views about whether they would or would not wish to receive active treatment should they suffer from certain conditions or illnesses. However, by their very nature, some conditions mean that those who have them may lack the physical or **cognitive** ability to communicate their wishes. For example, someone experiencing a stroke may not regain consciousness or a person with advanced dementia may be unable to communicate his or her wishes. Should active treatment be given in such circumstances, this could, if the individual were able to express his or her views, be experienced as abusive.

Recognising this situation, section 25 of the Mental Capacity Act makes provision for people to make an advance decision to refuse treatment while they have capacity in case they should lose capacity at a later date. This does not allow people to specify what treatment they do wish to receive, only to identify those interventions they do *not* wish to receive. To be valid the following criteria have to be met.

- It has to be made in writing.
- It has to be signed by the individual concerned or by someone else in his or her presence.
- It has to be witnessed by another person in his or her presence.
- It has to be verified by a statement by the person to whom the decision applies, stating that the decision is to apply even if life is at risk.

Having made an advanced decision, the individual concerned can change his or her mind at a later stage should he or she so wish.

Deprivation of liberty

Sometimes the behaviour of an individual can place him or her at risk of harm, for example someone with dementia who keeps wandering away from the ward. Such circumstances can be ethically challenging as, while we may not like the idea of depriving people of their liberty, this may be necessary to safeguard them from harm. The Deprivation of Liberty Safeguards make legal provision for this and provide a structure to safeguard both individuals at risk and those who provide care for them. To apply these safeguards individuals need to be assessed by two health and social care professionals to ensure that they lack decision-making capacity due to an impairment of the mind, that it is in their best interests to deprive them of their liberty, and that they would not be better protected under the provisions of the Mental Health Act 1983. Deprivation of liberty can be applied for a period of up to 12 months.

Ill-treatment and wilful neglect

The Mental Capacity Act 2005 makes provision for individuals to be prosecuted for either ill-treatment or neglect of someone who lacks capacity. To be prosecuted for ill-treatment a person needs to be found guilty of deliberately ill-treating someone or being reckless in that person's treatment. Examples might include someone deliberately hitting an individual because he or she has been incontinent, or causing someone psychological distress through 'teasing' him or her for the perpetrator's own amusement. In relation to neglect it has to be proven that someone deliberately failed to carry out an act that the person knew he or she had a duty to do. Examples here could include deliberately failing to provide someone with fluids or nutrition, or deliberately not checking to see if a person requires repositioning or changing in order to prevent pressure sores.

The inclusion of this provision in the Act is an important development as it allows for prosecution in some cases of abuse and neglect. However, since it only applies to people who lack capacity, there may be challenges to securing a conviction without clear evidence, which may be difficult to achieve where someone lacks capacity. In addition, it may not be a provision that people are aware of and so they may not know that seeking prosecution is an option.

Mental Health Act 1983

The main legislation relating to mental health in England and Wales is the Mental Health Act 1983 as amended by the Mental Health Act 2007. The implementation of this Act does, however, differ between England and Wales and each country has its own code relating to this legislation. Scotland has its own legislation and a link to the relevant webpage is included at the end of the chapter.

The provisions of this Act apply to those who are assessed as having a mental disorder that is defined as 'any disorder or disability of the mind', although a person with a learning disability can only be detained for treatment if his or her condition is accompanied by abnormally aggressive or seriously irresponsible conduct. The principles that underpin the Act include use of the least restrictive alternative, increased opportunities for review of **detention**, and multidisciplinary review.

In all instances the aim is for those suffering mental disorder and who require hospital treatment to do so on a voluntary basis. However, where the individual concerned refuses and he or she and/or others are at risk, compulsory admission may be necessary. Within the Act it is specified who can make an application for such an admission and who can authorise it, along with requirements in terms of duration and review. Table 6.2 provides brief details regarding the different sections that may be applied, although you are advised to consult the relevant website detailed at the end of the chapter for more information.

As you will have seen in Table 6.2, consent to treatment rules do not apply in all instances. This means that only those detained for the purposes of assessment and treatment may receive compulsory treatment under the direction of the approved clinician. Further safeguards are also in place in relation to treatments such as **psychosurgery**, treatments that include giving medication for a mental disorder beyond three months from when it was first prescribed, and **electroconvulsive therapy** (**ECT**). In these instances either the consent of the patient or the consent of an additional doctor is required.

Safeguards are included in relation to discharge from hospital. Community treatment orders allow detained patients to be discharged on the basis that they will be recalled to the hospital if they do not comply with treatment within a community setting. The Act also sets out a duty for health and social services to provide aftercare for as long as they feel is necessary for the patient. That this is stated as a 'duty' is positive in that it means it must be provided. However, it is up to services to decide how long it is necessary to provide such a service, which means that this could be open to interpretation especially in times of economic constraint.

Section	Duration	Application for review	Consent to treatment rules applicable
Section 4: Emergency admission for assessment	72 hours (but can be changed to another section if a second medical opinion is given during this period)	No	No
Section 2: Ordinary admission for assessment	28 days, not renewable	Yes, within the first 14 days	Yes
Section 3: Admission for assessment	6 months; can be renewed for 6 months and thereafter for 12 months	Yes, within the first 16 months	Yes
Section 5(2): Inpatient in hospital who appears to a registered medical practitioner to be in need of detention	72 hours, not renewable	No	No
Section 5 (4): Inpatient in hospital who appears to a nurse of a prescribed class to be in need of detention	6 hours, not renewable	No	No

Table 6.2 Mental Health Act 1983: key sections relating to compulsory admission

Equality Act 2010

Individuals and groups may be at risk of harm due to certain personal characteristics they have, or are thought to have. You will probably be familiar with the term 'discrimination' (see the glossary), which means that others are treated in a way that is unfair or unjust. To think about how this might occur within healthcare settings, and how it may lead to safeguarding concerns, take some time to read through the case studies below and then complete Activity 6.5.

Case study: Sally Carpenter

Sally Carpenter is a qualified nurse who has recently been moved to work on a medical ward that has a lot of older people admitted, sometimes for quite lengthy periods. Sally does not enjoy working with older people and believes that too many resources are wasted on them. Her manager has noticed that Sally tends to be very 'offhand' with older patients and often does not respond to their calls for assistance.

Case study: Peter Carmichael

Peter Carmichael is 26 years old and has severe learning disabilities and complex health needs. He has been very unwell recently and has been admitted to hospital with a severe respiratory infection. While in A&E with Peter, his parents are told that 'normally' admission to the intensive therapy unit would take place, but that in 'cases like Peter's' the medical team do not feel this is appropriate and they would like to discuss whether active treatment should be given.

Case study: Hilary Parsons

Hilary Parsons is 45 years old and has a history of bipolar disorder. When her mood is depressed she is known to self-harm, but she usually manages to tell someone and receives appropriate treatment. During her current period of depression she has contacted her primary care team indicating that she feels she is going to self-harm; however, her telephone calls have not been followed up because she had previously threatened this and had not carried it out. Hilary was found later having taken an overdose and, on admission to A&E, was treated in a very dismissive way because the staff felt she only had herself to blame and that they should be free to treat people who are really sick.

Activity 6.5   *Critical thinking*

Look at each of the above case studies and decide whether you feel an individual or a group of individuals was treated unfairly.

- Why do you feel they were treated unfairly?
- What safeguarding concerns can you identify?
- Think about your own practice – have you ever come across situations where you feel people have been discriminated against?

Outline answers are given at the end of the chapter.

Unfortunately, in answering the questions in Activity 6.5, you will probably have identified situations where discrimination has occurred. Given that such treatment is unfair and unjust, and can give rise to safeguarding concerns, it is important that measures are taken to safeguard against it.

In October 2010 the Equality Act came into force to simplify existing provisions by bringing together over one hundred pieces of legislation within one Act. It aims to protect individuals from discrimination and to promote a fairer and more equitable society. It includes a range of measures such as strengthening the protection provided for disabled people and requiring **reasonable adjustments** to be made to accommodate disabled people. It also aims to protect people from discrimination by association or by perception: this means that it is illegal to discriminate against someone because he or she is believed to have a particular characteristic or because (for example) he or she is the parent or partner of someone who has a particular characteristic or condition. For instance, it would not be legal to discriminate against someone who has a mental health problem or because he or she is *thought* to have a mental health problem. Similarly, it would not be acceptable to discriminate against the parents of a disabled child while they are seeking employment because it is assumed that they will need to take a lot of time off work.

Within the Act a Single Public Sector Equality Duty is specified and this identifies the various grounds on which discrimination must not occur:

- age;
- disability;
- gender reassignment;
- pregnancy and maternity;
- race;
- religion and belief;
- sex;
- sexual orientation.

To support implementation of the Act, the Equalities Commission has produced a range of guides and background information. Take some time to visit its website (given at the end of the chapter) to find out more about the Act.

Confidentiality

Usually, upholding confidentiality is viewed as an essential aspect of professional nursing care. However, what if a patient who has a mental health problem tells you that he or she is being sexually abused but doesn't want you to tell anyone? What if you visit a family at home with your mentor and you observe that an adult with learning disabilities is being emotionally abused? You raise the issue with your mentor but he or she says that what the family tells you must be kept confidential. The professional issues are discussed further in Chapter 7, but here the legal implications are briefly discussed.

As Griffith and Tengnah (2010) argue, *Neither the professional nor legal duties of confidentiality are absolute and they are subject to a range of exceptions that justify disclosure* (p202). They observe, however, that the

Code (NMC, 2008a) leaves decisions regarding disclosure to the professional judgement of nurses, although inappropriate breach of confidence would be viewed as professional misconduct.

In the context of safeguarding, there can be ethical dilemmas as you have to weigh the consequences of sharing information and the consequences of not sharing information. Read the scenario below and then the two possible courses of action and their outcomes.

Scenario: Mrs Thompson

Imagine you are a district nurse who visits a patient, Mrs Thompson, who is an older person, lives alone and has limited mobility. She says that her daughter sees to her needs, but one day when you visit you find the flat very cold and you ask Mrs Thompson if the heating has broken down. She replies that her daughter can't afford to pay the gas bill. You get her to talk more about her daughter and it emerges that she takes all of Mrs Thompson's money, bringing her a few groceries each week. She says, however, that she doesn't want you to tell anyone. What should you do?

Option 1*: You leave feeling very concerned but decide to do as you have been asked and not tell anyone. A few days later you come into work to find that Mrs Thompson has been admitted due to a fall and hypothermia. She has also been found to have a very poor nutritional status.*

Option 2*: You leave feeling very concerned both about Mrs Thompson and about your own position. You decide to talk through the case with your manager and you both agree that there seems to be financial abuse occurring. You contact the identified lead for vulnerable adults who visits Mrs Thompson. Initially, she is distressed that you have told someone but then admits to feeling relieved as she was scared of her daughter and didn't feel able to challenge her alone.*

You have a dilemma – you feel torn between your duty to respect confidentiality and a professional responsibility to raise your concerns with someone. Not breaking confidentiality can, however, have negative consequences and we need to remember that disclosing suspected abuse without the consent of the patient is allowed in certain circumstances (DH, 2003, 2010c).

Barriers to implementation of policy and legislation

The existence of policies and legislation does not guarantee their implementation: barriers may occur. Think back to Activity 6.3 – how aware were people you asked of their human rights? If, for example, people do not know that they have a right to freedom from torture, they may accept treatment that is physically or psychologically damaging because they do not know that it is prohibited and that it can be challenged. Similarly, while it is to be hoped that everyone knows it is morally wrong to torture another person, some individuals may not know that other people have a legal right to freedom from torture. In both of these cases the impact of the Human Rights

Act 1998 will be limited due to a lack of awareness. Policies and laws will only be implemented if people are aware of them.

Sometimes people and/or organisations are aware of policies and laws but they lack the commitment to implement them. Examples of this include situations where an organisation fails to provide the training necessary to enable staff to understand their responsibilities within a policy. Similarly, individuals or groups of staff may be aware of a new policy but may either decide not to find out more about it or choose not to comply. Sometimes policy may be issued in the form of guidance rather than being binding, and therefore individuals and organisations are free to choose not to follow such guidance. Take some time to complete Activity 6.6 to see how this works.

Activity 6.6　　　　　　　　　　　　　　　　　　　　*Critical thinking*

Look at the following statements that might appear in a policy statement concerning safeguarding.

* All agencies should consider the use of systems to record reports of abuse.
* All agencies have a duty to develop, implement and monitor common systems of recording allegations of abuse.

What do you think are the important differences between these two statements? What difference would they make in practice?

Some possible implications are discussed at the end of this chapter.

How policy and legislation are worded can have a significant effect on how they are implemented. This can have a significant impact on whether the policy or legislation is seen as a priority and whether resources are committed to supporting its implementation. Resources in this context can include staffing, equipment, buildings and time and, while some policies can be implemented within existing resources, this is not always the case; when finances are stretched priorities have to be set, and not all demands are met. Unless policies require action they may not be viewed as a priority and resources may not be committed to support their implementation.

Nursing practice, safeguarding and legislation

This book is concerned with supporting you in understanding your role in safeguarding adults and it is important to stress the links between legislation and policy, and the role of the nurse. As has been discussed above, one barrier to policy implementation is a lack of awareness and it is important that all nurses are aware of the key policy and legal provisions relevant to their areas of work. To help you think about this, take some time to complete Activity 6.7.

Activity 6.7 — *Leadership and management*

Take a look at the table below and try to identify, for each clinical setting, some of the key policies and legislation of which you would need to be aware if you were working there.

Clinical setting	Relevant legislation and policy
An acute medical ward that regularly has older people with dementia admitted	
An acute mental inpatient unit	
An assessment and treatment unit for people with learning disabilities	
A nursing home that provides care for a mix of older frail people with a range of needs	

Some suggestions are provided at the end of the chapter.

In Activity 6.7 you will have seen that there are some key policies and legislation that nurses need to be aware of if they are to safeguard adults wherever they work. This book has provided you with an introduction to these, but this is an area of knowledge you will need continually to review and extend. At the end of this chapter you will find some suggestions for further reading and websites that will help you with this.

Being aware of the broad provisions within policy and legislation is, however, only the first step towards safeguarding: you also need to recognise when it is relevant to use it and how it can be applied to safeguarding individual patients and clients.

Case study: Mr Waters

You are a newly qualified nurse working in a medical ward where Mr Waters, who is 84, is admitted with pneumonia. Due to breathlessness, Mr Waters finds it very difficult to speak, but he draws the attention of staff to a document that is an advance decision to refuse treatment, stating that should he contract pneumonia he does not wish to be treated with antibiotics even if this results in his death. The document has been witnessed by a solicitor. The admitting doctor spoke with Mr Waters about the document and asked him if

continued . . .

this was still his wish: he nodded, indicating agreement. A decision was taken to just provide him with palliative care but to check regularly if he had changed his mind. His daughter, who lives a considerable distance away, has come to visit her father and is very distressed to find that he is not being actively treated. She accuses the hospital of ageism and demands that he is given antibiotics immediately. How would you respond to Mr Waters' daughter?

In this case study it is likely that a nurse having a good understanding of the Mental Capacity Act 2005 would have greater confidence in responding to Mr Waters' daughter. This is not to deny the fact that explaining his decision would be challenging, but rather to suggest that if you are confident that you have a good knowledge base it is easier to present a coherent argument. This highlights the needs for nurses to be aware of the legislation and policy relevant to safeguarding the patients and clients with whom they work. If you think about dealing with fires, you would find it very strange if you were told 'We don't have a fire procedure, we just wait until it happens and then go and look up what we need to know.' The same is true of legislation and policy – it is better to think ahead and be prepared.

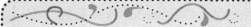

Chapter summary

This chapter has explored policy and legislation by examining the process through which they are developed and implemented, and then by discussing some key areas of policy relevant to safeguarding. Barriers to implementation were considered and the importance of nurses having both knowledge of key legislation, and an understanding of how to apply it in practice, was stressed. However, it is important to remember that policy and legislation are constantly evolving and it is necessary to be aware of sources of information that can be used to keep up to date. The web addresses at the end of this chapter are a good starting point and you may also wish to visit your local health and social services web pages to check out local policies and procedures.

Activities: Brief outline answers

Activity 6.1 Decision making, page 109

It might have shocked you to read that, even though policies were in place, this situation was able to occur. You might also have thought about what you would have done in this situation – you might find it helpful to read the NMC (2010b) publication *Raising and Escalating Concerns* for further advice here.

Activity 6.2 Critical thinking, page 110

In undertaking this activity you may have found it challenging to think of areas where human rights may be infringed within healthcare settings. However, when you start to consider the various rights, it soon becomes clear how easy it is for rights not to be upheld in practice. Indeed, a number of high-profile cases have been cited in the media recently as examples of how rights have been infringed – treatment provided in an inhumane manner, basic needs such as nutrition and hydration not met, and even situations where premature death has occurred. It is also possible to recognise other situations that are unlikely to lead to cases being brought under the Human Rights Act 1998, but that nonetheless provide evidence of rights not being upheld. These include a lack of privacy, and not treating people with respect.

Activity 6.3 Reflection, page 111

While it is impossible to comment on the extent to which the people you asked were aware of their rights under the Human Rights Act 1998, it is unlikely that everyone was able to name all of them accurately. Some people may not even have been aware that they had such rights. This is likely to be true of many of the patients and families you work with, particularly those who have dementia, learning disabilities or mental health problems. This reduces the extent to which they are safeguarded as they cannot defend rights they do not know they possess. Others (including nurses) may need to advocate on their behalf.

Activity 6.4 Communication, page 112

Staff observed Luke's behaviour and his lack of verbal communication and immediately jumped to the conclusion that he had mental health problems or a learning disability. This was reinforced by his 'aggression', which they interpreted as further evidence. However, knowing he had an allergy, seeing the syringe and not having a way of communicating his concerns make his behaviour seem a reasonable response to his situation. This activity highlights the importance of trying differing ways of communicating with people when seeking consent to treatment and of not making assumptions about capacity. It also highlights how nurses can support individuals to safeguard themselves by (for example) always carrying a card providing emergency information.

Activity 6.5 Critical thinking, page 117

Discrimination and prejudice are evident in each of these case studies, where people are treated less favourably because of age, learning disabilities and mental health problems. Assumptions are held about them based on certain characteristics and, because of this, they are seen to be of less worth than other people and/or to have a poorer quality of life. In some instances this behaviour can be very visible, such as in the first and third case studies. In others (such as the second case study) it can be more subtle, where judgements concerning quality of life are implied but never actually stated.

Activity 6.6 Critical thinking, page 120

The key difference between these two policy statements is that the first recommends a course of action but does not require such action to be taken. It leaves room for discretion. In contrast, the second statement imposes a duty on agencies to undertake a range of actions and requires collaboration to ensure that recording systems are common. You might find it interesting to look at some examples of both national and local policies to see how they are worded and what the implications are.

Activity 6.7 Leadership and management, page 121

Some legislation is relevant to each of these areas, such as the Human Rights Act 1998 and the Mental Capacity Act 2005. Similarly, policies relating to safeguarding/protection of vulnerable adults will apply in each setting. Others, such as the Mental Health Act 1983, will, however, more likely be relevant to mental health settings, and the assessment and treatment unit for people with learning disabilities.

Further reading

Dimond, B (2008) *Legal Aspects of Mental Capacity*. Oxford: Blackwell.

This is a useful text for deepening and extending your understanding of the Mental Capacity Act 2005.

Griffith, R and Tengnah, C (2010) *Law and Professional Issues in Nursing*, 2nd edition. Exeter: Learning Matters.

This is a useful introduction to legal aspects of nursing that includes sections relevant to safeguarding.

Herring, J (2010) *Medical Law and Ethics*. Oxford: Oxford University Press.

This is a more in-depth text that covers a range of legal and ethical issues including capacity, consent, confidentiality and mental health law.

Mandelstam, M (2009) *Safeguarding Vulnerable Adults and the Law*. London: Jessica Kingsley.

This is a good overview of key legislation relating to safeguarding adults.

Useful websites

www.cqc.org.uk/public

This is the website of the Care Quality Commission, which inspects care provision within England.

www.dh.gov.uk/en/Publicationsandstatistics/Publications/PublicationsPolicyAndGuidance/DH_084597

This provides access to the *Code of Practice* for the Mental Capacity Act.

www.equalityhumanrights.com

This is the website of the Equality and Human Rights Commission, giving specific information regarding the Human Rights Act as well as wider information regarding rights.

www.justice.gov.uk

This contains information concerning the Mental Capacity Act and its *Code of Practice*.

www.legislation.gov.uk

This site enables you to search for any UK, Welsh, Scottish or Northern Irish legislation.

The following three sites provide information concerning legislation and policy in Wales, Northern Ireland and Scotland:

http://wales.gov.uk/?skip=1&lang=en

www.niassembly.gov.uk

www.scotland.gov.uk/Topics

Chapter 7
Professional frameworks

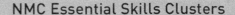

NMC Essential Skills Clusters

This chapter will address the following ESCs:

Cluster: Care, compassion and communication

6.   People can trust the newly registered graduate nurse to protect and keep as confidential all information relating to them.

Cluster: Organisational aspects of care

19.   People can trust the newly registered graduate nurse to work to prevent and resolve conflict and maintain a safe environment.

Chapter aims

By the end of this chapter you should be able to:

*   discuss the purpose and functions of a professional code of conduct related to nursing;
*   identify the different stages of raising concerns in the workplace and when it would be appropriate to blow the whistle;
*   discuss the main elements of clinical supervision and how they relate to safeguarding;
*   recognise the implications for nursing practice.

Introduction

Nursing is viewed as a profession and as such the public will expect each individual member to act and behave in a professional manner. The Nursing and Midwifery Council (NMC) sets out the standards expected of the nurse with regard to values, behaviour, competence, knowledge and skills. Sometimes some nurses fall short of these ideals and are therefore subject to a range of sanctions. The aims of this chapter are therefore to critically review the implications of professional codes in relation to safeguarding and protecting the public. It also aims to explore the difficulties with raising concerns regarding abuse and poor practice as well as considering strategies for practice development such as clinical supervision and reflective practice.

Codes of conduct

Before reading further, try Activity 7.1.

Activity 7.1   *Critical thinking*

Consider carefully the following questions.

- Define what is meant by a profession; can you identify the key elements that you would expect to see in a definition of a profession?
- What is a code of conduct and how does it link to a profession?
- What are the functions of codes of conduct?

There is no outline answer at the end of the chapter. Instead, compare your ideas with the information given below.

There is no standard definition of a profession as it is difficult to get universal agreement. However, a number of important elements of what would constitute a profession are contained in the Professions Australia (2004) definition of a profession as:

[a] disciplined group of individuals who adhere to ethical standards and who hold themselves out as, and are accepted by the public as, possessing special knowledge and skills in a widely recognised body of learning derived from research, education and training at a high level, and who are prepared to apply this knowledge and exercise these skills in the interest of others. It is inherent in the definition of a profession that a code of ethics governs the activities of each profession.

Many different groups of people may lay claim to being a profession, for example nurses, social workers, police officers, engineers, firemen, estate agents or accountants. Nursing has only relatively recently established itself as a profession by building up its research base and moving away from nurses being seen as the handmaidens of doctors. Many highly skilled nurses are undertaking procedures that were previously the sole responsibility of medical staff, such as prescribing medicines, taking bloods and some minor surgical procedures. So we can see that the key elements of a profession are:

- having highly skilled and disciplined members;
- having a strong research base that informs education and training;
- having members who have undertaken specialised training and obtained qualifications;
- being recognised by the general public as a profession;
- being prepared to serve the public;
- having a code of ethics or conduct to regulate the behaviour of professionals.

One of the main elements of a profession is therefore a code of conduct with an ethical dimension (see Chapter 3). In order for the public to acknowledge and have confidence in a professional group of individuals, they expect them to behave properly and to a high standard. One way of doing this is to have a code of behaviour or conduct and some ethical guidance to help with decision making. For example, the public would not expect police officers to break the

Function	Explanation
Ethical	A code should influence the professional in ethical decision making by stressing important elements. For example, in nursing this would be putting the patient/client first.
Guidance	A code should be able to offer professionals guidance on their duties and obligations in practice.
Discipline	Professionals will be held accountable for the actions and their code will be used to judge them if they act unprofessionally. The code therefore acts to regulate the profession.
Protection	A code offers some reassurance to the public that standards have been set for professionals and if they act 'unprofessionally' they may lose their professional status. The public should be able to trust professionals to do their best for them.
Political	A code often spells out a set of ideals and aspirations that the professional should always strive to meet. Professionals can use their codes to fight for better standards.
Competence	A code should require professionals to keep up to date with their knowledge and skills. The public would expect professionals to be proficient and skilful in carrying out their practice.

Table 7.1 Functions of professional codes

law and nurses to harm and abuse people in their care. There are a number of functions that codes perform – see Table 7.1 for some examples.

Unfortunately, no professional code of conduct, including those codes with an ethical dimension, can tell you what to do in every given situation. In spite of this, codes are useful guides and, even if on their own they cannot solve ethical dilemmas, they can influence the decisions taken by nurses. However, Tadd (1994) questions the usefulness of professional codes to empower practitioners and asks whether nurses would actually notice if their *Code* disappeared overnight. This is due in part to its lack of support for nurses who uphold some of its principles, particularly those who blow the whistle. Pattison and Wainwright (2010) go further and argue that the current *Code* (NMC, 2008a) is not really a code of ethics as it lacks clear ethical guidance.

Activity 7.2 — *Reflection and critical thinking*

First obtain a couple of copies of different professional codes of conduct via the internet. Some may be more difficult to access and obtain than others and you will need to reflect on some of the possible reasons and implications of this. Some of the most common codes of conduct can be obtained from the following websites.

Nursing: www.nmc-uk.org/Documents/Standards/The-code-A4–20100406.pdf

Social care workers: www.gscc.org.uk/cmsFiles/CodesofPracticeforSocialCareWorkers.pdf

Registered teachers: http://dera.ioe.ac.uk/11660/2/code_of_conduct_1009.pdf

Once you have obtained copies, compare and contrast the main elements of each with the NMC *Code*. Answer the following questions.

- What are the differences and similarities between the codes?
- Do you think the public, especially vulnerable adults, would be able to understand what the NMC *Code* means?
- For the NMC *Code* – Can you identify the various functions of codes (listed in Table 7.1) within this specific code of ethics?
- Do you think it would help you with ethical dilemmas? (Revisit Chapter 3, which focuses on ethics and will be particularly helpful to you.)
- What are the main safeguarding elements of this code?

See the outline answers at the end of this chapter for further guidance on the last two questions.

On reflection, you would think that the general public should have easy access to any professional code and should be able to obtain a copy with minimal fuss. Professional bodies should ensure ease of availability and make their codes accessible for those with disabilities or whose main language is not English. The NMC website, www.nmc-uk.org, is a good example of this in some aspects. This is in areas such as free publications in different formats, a general public website, feedback and accessibility windows; also, the site is relatively easy to navigate around and consideration is given to other languages. You may have found other professional codes were more difficult to locate.

In terms of similarities and differences between codes, you might have found that codes have a series of statements of standards of behaviour. These may relate to putting adults or children first, treating people with respect and dignity, working together, upholding public trust, protection and maintaining high standards. There will be differences depending on the nature of the profession. For example, the code for social workers places more explicit emphasis on social issues, such as inclusion, diversity, fairness, power and justice, whereas the NMC *Code* places more emphasis on health issues.

Many of the functions of codes, highlighted in Table 7. 1, can be seen in the NMC *Code*.

The statement, *Failure to comply with this code may bring your fitness to practise into question and endanger your registration,* indicates the disciplinary function. In this statement – *You must act without delay if you believe that you, a colleague or anyone else may be putting someone at risk* – you can see the protective function. Some functions are less obvious and, if you examine the following statement – *You must inform someone in authority if you experience problems that prevent you working within this code or other nationally agreed standards* – you may be forgiven in thinking that it has just a guidance and a protective function. However, it also serves a political function in that you can use it to argue for more resources in order to meet such national standards. For example, you may find low staffing levels have a negative impact on the time you spend safeguarding vulnerable adults as you have to undertake additional duties.

Addressing professional misconduct and fitness to practise

The NMC believes that a nurse's suitability to be on its professional register requires a practitioner to meet the following requirements:

- *achieving the standards of proficiency required for entry to and maintenance on the register;*
- *the maintenance of good health and good character to enable safe and effective practice;*
- *adherence to the principles of good practice set out in the code and other guidance provided by the NMC.*
(2011, p4)

Sadly, professionals on occasions fall well below the standards expected of them by their peers and the general public. When they do this they can be reported to their professional bodies and, in the case of registered nurses, this will be to the NMC. Any person, organisation and service can report a registered nurse to the NMC. The police have a legal requirement to report registered nurses to the NMC if they have been cautioned for or convicted of a criminal offence. Ideally, concerns should be raised with the nurse's employer first and often the problem can be dealt with at this level. However, allegations sometimes need to be referred to the NMC and it can be seen on Table 7.2 that employers most frequently refer nurses to the NMC. Reporting by colleagues makes up a small percentage and it is evident that the general public are increasingly ready to report potential misconduct.

Source of referral	Number of referrals	Percentage
Employers	1,743	41
Police	909	23
Public	915	23
Self, solicitors, educational institutions, colleagues	495	13
Anonymous	110	4
Other medical professionals	39	2

Table 7.2 Referral figures (NMC, 2011, p18)

Although misconduct makes up a large percentage of complaints, fitness to practise can also be impaired by other factors such as lack of competence, physical or mental health problems or drug or alcohol abuse. Good health is an essential part of fitness to practise, although that should not preclude nurses with disabilities or long-term health problems. You can still practise safely and competently with and without adjustments being made in the workplace. Problems usually arise when a nurse does not acknowledge that he or she has a health problem or may be abusing alcohol and drugs. The responsibility is on the practitioner to sort themselves out and not to put others at risk. The types of allegations made against registered nurses and midwives are identified in Table 7.3, although it must be remembered that many of the cases involve more than one type of allegation.

Nature of allegations made	Examples	Percentage
Dishonesty	• theft • obtaining goods by deception	25
Competency issues	• maladministration of drugs • neglect of basic care	24
Patients	• verbal/physical/sexual abuse • inappropriate relationships with patients	22
Other practice-related issues	• unsafe clinical practice	7
Other	• convictions	5
Record keeping	• failure to maintain adequate records	4
Violence	• convictions • patient abuse	4
Pornography	• child pornography	4
Colleagues	• failure to co-operate with colleagues • physical, verbal or sexual abuse • inappropriate relationships	3
Substance misuse	• illicit drugs • alcohol	3
Serious motoring offences	• theft of a vehicle	2
Drugs	• maladministration • theft of drugs	2
Management practices	• unsafe clinical practice • failure to collaborate with colleagues	2 2

Table 7.3 Types of allegation considered by the Conduct and Competence Committee in 2010–11 (NMC, 2011, pp20–1)

On the NMC website, www.nmc-uk.org, under the 'Hearings' window, you will find a monthly list of nurses who are appearing before the various committees and also the outcomes. Reflect on whether you think this is a good or bad thing and then answer the following questions.

- Do you think the sanctions were appropriate in relation to the nature of the charges? You will need to find out the range of sanctions.
- Is it right that a fellow nurse and members of the public can attend such hearings?
- How would you feel if your name appeared on this site if your practice was called into question?

See the outline answers at the end of this chapter for some direction in formulating your ideas.

Raising concerns and whistle-blowing

Read the following scenario and then attempt Activity 7.4.

Scenario: Bad practice – to tell or not to tell?

As a student or registered nurse you are working on a new placement. You have to receive a positive evaluation for your time spent there from your mentor. On your first and other days you witness some poor practice – staff ignoring patients' requests for help, hoists and other safety equipment not being used, meals being missed and some medication being administered late or not at all. At the end of the week you mention this to your mentor during the supervision session. Your mentor sighs, rolls her eyes upwards and puts her finger to her lips. She tells you that this is normal practice as this is a very busy placement and to forget what they tell you in college as they haven't a clue what goes on currently in practice. She also suggests that, to get a good report, you must keep your head down and just get on with things 'like in her day'. She then tells you that you are doing really well and the patients love you. You discuss what you have witnessed with a colleague who is on placement with you and he tells you the area is fine and is one of the better placements.

Imagine you were the student on the placement in the above scenario.

- How do you feel you would react in such a situation?
- Would you also raise your concerns with your mentor knowing that potentially it could impact on your final report?
- Would you be satisfied with such a response from your mentor?
- If you were not satisfied with the response, what else do you feel you should do?

Answers will be provided in the following text.

All nurses will have their own reasons, personal to them, on why they do or do not speak out. Nurses have a professional responsibility to speak out if abuse is suspected. This should be a straightforward action but you may feel that you are being pressured to keep silent on the matter. This is done by the mentor in the above scenario, who, far from being supportive, attempts to justify the actions of staff by referring to the area as being busy. The mentor also implies that, in order to get a good report, it is advisable not to 'rock the boat'. This is clear not only through what the mentor says but how she says it. **Non-verbal communication** can be very powerful and gestures such as eye-rolling can be very dismissive and make you feel that you are also wasting her time. One potential area of difficulty is that you are a lone voice, as nobody else seems to have witnessed the same events as you or, if they have, they have chosen to say silent. This should not put you off reporting and, if the mentor does nothing, you should take your observations to the next level. After all, at this stage you are only raising concerns about suspected abuse or poor practice and nothing has been proven. Getting a good report or gaining personal credit is always secondary to the needs of patients/clients as the care of people is your first concern (NMC, 2008a).

Firtko and Jackson have defined whistle-blowing as *the reporting of information to an individual, group or body that is not part of the organisation's usual problem-solving strategy* (2005, p52). Making the decision to blow the whistle when you feel that nobody is taking notice of your concerns is very difficult. This is particularly the case in nursing as many friendships are formed and it can be a very close-knit community. The fear of potential repercussions, such as colleagues not speaking to you, being abused or not being considered for promotions, can make individuals think twice about speaking out (Manthorpe and Stanley, 1999). A study by Ahern and McDonald (2002) reviewed the literature, to explore the beliefs that might act as motivational factors for nurses to decide to blow the whistle or to keep silent. They found that whistle-blowers identified more strongly with beliefs based on the principles of advocacy and believed they were more responsible to their patients above everything else. Non-whistle-blowers tended to side more with the wishes and responsibilities of doctors and employers in balance with responsibilities to the patient.

The high-profile cases highlighted in Chapter 1 of nurses Graham Pink, Margaret Haywood and Terry Bryan (see page 21 and Activity 1.7) illustrate the consequences of blowing the whistle, which may put people off doing so. The short- and long-term effects on the individual can be very profound, sometimes leading to dismissal. In Chapter 1 it has already been discussed that, where one nurse whistle-blower stands up, there are many other potential whistle-blowers who have chosen to remain silent. There may be many personal and professional reasons why nurses have held back from their professional responsibilities. Some of these reasons may relate to the type of environment or culture they are working in.

Activity 7.5 — Critical thinking

In the above discussion, some of the reasons for not speaking out or blowing the whistle have been highlighted. Now consider carefully the factors that need to be in place in order for nurses to feel confident in speaking out in cases of suspected abuse, so that there would be no need to blow the whistle.

An answer will be provided in the following text.

Let us take one step back and remember that, if an organisation has competent staff, suitable environments and good care practices, it is more likely to have fewer concerns regarding abusive practices and general complaints. As well as creating empowering environments for patients/clients, it is equally important to empower staff (Jenkins, 1997). Therefore, having a working environment that has the factors shown in Table 7.4 is helpful in fostering a culture of openness whereby concerns can be raised without fear.

Whistle-blowing is protected by law with the Public Interest Disclosure Act 1998 creating a system of support across the private, public and voluntary sectors. It protects workers who blow the

Factor	Requirements
Complaints procedure	Needs to be supported by staff by being current, regularly reviewed and effective, with outcomes leading to improvements. Needs to include whistle-blowing.
Safeguarding policies	Policies are increasingly referring directly to the idea of thresholds (see section 'Thresholds and decision making' in Chapter 4, pages 70–2) and are providing guidance on making the decision about whether a situation requires a response via **POVA** or an alternative response. Clear guidance and regular discussions need to be in place and undertaken.
Open culture	Staff and clients must be able to raise concerns without fear of repercussions.
Clinical supervision	This must be regular and confidential, ideally with an independent supervisor to facilitate sessions.
Reflective practice	Nurses should be encouraged to reflect on their practice, particularly when they have concerns regarding speaking out about abuse.
Staff training	This should help develop staff with assertiveness, confidence in dealing with criticism and concerns, competence levels and safeguarding. Staff should explore areas such as thresholds for action and what is good, bad and abusive practice.
Person-centred care	This approach should ensure that control remains with the client and should instil the values of dignity and respect for all.
Advocacy	Promoting the use of independent advocacy services for clients without external support.

Table 7.4 Factors for a suitable working environment for nurses

whistle about wrongdoing and it applies where a worker has a reasonable belief that their disclosure tends to show one or more of the following offences or breaches:

- criminal offences;
- failure to comply with a legal obligation;
- miscarriages of justice;
- threats to health and safety;
- damage to the environment;
- deliberate covering up of information (any of the above).

(See the Direct.gov website at www.direct.gov.uk or the Health and Safety Executive website at www.hse.gov.uk.)

Staff awareness raising and training in what to do if they have concerns are crucial prerequisites to staff feeling confident to blow the whistle. They need to have clarity on what their professional responsibilities are. The NMC, in response to this, issued specific guidance for nurses on raising and escalating concerns. See Figure 7.1 for the five stages of this process.

The NMC is strongly suggesting that raising concerns externally, especially whistle-blowing, should only ever be undertaken after careful consideration of all the issues and when all the internal complaints procedures have been exhausted. In a nutshell, this means that all the avenues should have been explored internally, and externally to regulatory bodies (stage 4), and that there was nowhere else to go, except to the public (stage 5).

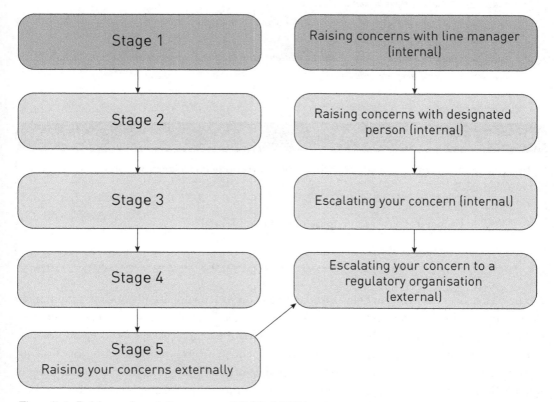

Figure 7.1 Raising and escalating concerns (NMC, 2010b)

Confidentiality

During your time in nursing you will come across many situations where you will have access to personal and sensitive information. In some situations you can openly discuss issues, while in others there will be a need to keep information confidential. The legal and ethical implications of confidentiality were discussed in the previous chapter. The NMC (2009) states that a *duty of confidence arises when one person discloses information to another in circumstances where it is reasonable to expect that the information will be held in confidence.* In nursing, there will be many such situations whereby patients will give you information, expecting it to be used only for the purpose for which it is given. For example, it would be reasonable for you to expect a patient to disclose to you how often he or she went to the toilet if you were carrying out an assessment for a urinary tract infection. The patient would, in turn, reasonably expect you to use this information in deciding what treatment plan you developed. However, the patient would not expect it to be used as part of a clinical trial for a new drug, if he or she were not first made aware of this and had not been asked for permission. The patient would certainly not expect this information to be shared with one of the cleaners on the ward or a visitor. Essentially, patients/clients provide nurses with information because they put their *trust* in nurses to use such information appropriately and to respect their wishes.

The NMC *Code* reminds nurses that they:

- *must respect people's right to confidentiality;*
- *must ensure people are informed about how and why information is shared by those who will be providing their care;*
- *must disclose information if [they] believe someone may be at risk of harm, in line with the law of the country in which [they] are practising.*

(2008a, p3)

Activity 7.6   *Reflection*

Imagine an environment or society where there was no need to keep personal information confidential.

- What would this be like?
- Why do we need to keep some information confidential?

Answers will be provided in the following text.

You may have been surprised at being asked to reflect on such an apparently obvious requirement as to keep some information confidential. However, sometimes it is necessary to take a step back and reflect on why we do the things we do, particularly the actions we see as accepted practice. The clear advantage of having an open environment in which information is free flowing, without restrictions, is that there is more of a chance of developing a greater understanding of individuals' needs and situations. In some close-knit communities, strong bonds form and there is a comradeship in which people help each other. Free-flowing information is necessary for the community to help individuals when they fall into difficulty and are in need of support. Some healthcare environments can become like this, such as in intensive and palliative care. Interestingly, these types of environments tend to have fewer reports of abusive practices taking place. However, it may be frustrating at times for some individuals as it may seem that everyone knows everyone else's business. In a sense, we are socialised into accepting or not accepting the free flow of information.

However, it is not just the way we are socialised into being open or restricted in our everyday discussions. The law is clear: the Human Rights Act 1998, article 8, states that *everyone has the right to respect for his private and family life, his home and his correspondence.* There are also provisions in common law and in the statutes that respect the right of UK citizens to have personal information kept confidential (the law is discussed in more detail in Chapter 6).

Activity 7.7   *Reflection and critical thinking*

Consider the following three scenarios.

Scenario 1: A close work colleague confesses to you on an evening out that he lied on the application form to work on your unit, which specialises in working with young adults who have been sexually abused. The job advert made clear in the essential criteria that the candidate must possess a psychotherapy qualification and must have had the post-qualifying experience of counselling victims of abuse. Your work colleague said he used his wife's qualification as they both share the same name – Sam Harris. He said he worked with her counselling victims in the past and that, in fact, he had taught her all she knew but was not very good at passing exams. He also tells you he is in a lot of debt and needed the extra money.

Scenario 2: A terminally ill woman you are nursing confesses to you that her son James, who comes in to visit her on a regular basis, is not the biological son of her husband. This was the result of an affair when she lived in Tanzania. James has looked after her for the last ten years, sacrificing his career to do this. Her husband, Leroy, has only visited her once and then it was to demand money from her to pay for a holiday for himself. The woman wants you to tell James the truth but only after her death. She does not want Leroy to know as she fears that he will hurt or disown James.

Scenario 3: You are covering for your manager and have to access his computer. On going through his files you come across a file of images of famous landmarks and instructions on how to put together explosive devices. Your manager is well known for having radical views on a range of political topics.

- Reflect on how you would initially feel in each of these scenarios.
- What would be the issues you would need to consider in each of these situations?
- What would be the eventual course of action that you would take in terms of confidentiality?

Answers will be provided in the following text.

In terms of reflecting on all three scenarios you might feel in each a sense of 'why me?' Why have you been put in this situation or stumbled across this dilemma? In the first and second scenarios, why have people confided in you with their secrets and is there an expectation that you will keep them? Is it also that they have total trust in you to keep quiet or carry out their wishes? In the third scenario, you may feel surprised, horrified or very alarmed, depending on the nature of the relationship you have with your line manager or how you view such a risk to the public.

In scenario 1 it is clear that your work colleague obtained the post by deception. You may have some sympathy for him due to his financial situation and because he is a close work colleague. However, he is now working, without the necessary skills and qualifications, with vulnerable people who have suffered from abuse. Therefore, potentially his interventions may be harmful to individuals attempting to recover from their abuse. He also potentially puts organisations and colleagues at risk if he does not have the required level of competence. In some employment situations he may be breaking the law if he claimed he had a particular professional status such as a registered nursing qualification. Ideally, you would try to encourage the individual to own up to his employers that he did not have the qualifications and necessary experience to undertake this type of sensitive work. You would also insist that he stopped all therapy until he did own up and that you would report him if he did not. The timescale would be very short for doing this, and this is one type of confidence that you would not want to keep, as your first concern would be to clients.

In scenario 2, you may have a great deal of sympathy for both the woman involved and her son. You may be less sympathetic for her husband as, on the face of it, he has not been very supportive. However, nurses caring for individuals only ever have a snapshot in time and often only the perspective of the individual they are caring for. You will not have the history of each of the people involved, their relationship to each other or how they each view their own situation. Again, as in scenario 1, it would be best to try to get the mother to talk to her son or get her to confide in a family friend. There is a potential here to create more distress for all concerned. You would need to seek advice from your line manager and professional organisation or trade union. A duty to the patient is still owed even after death (NMC, 2009), so you need to be careful.

In the third and final scenario, you would need to think very carefully before you act. You have some suspicions and also some evidence. As it is your line manager's computer, you will need to report your observations/findings to a more senior manager. The NMC (2009) highlights that there are some particular situations when the law allows confidentiality to be broken. The following laws place a duty on individuals to undertake certain actions:

- Public Health Act 1984 – duty to report a notifiable disease;
- Public Health (Infectious Diseases) Regulations 1998 – duty to report relevant infectious diseases;
- Road Traffic Act 1998 – duty to report to the police, when questioned, the name and address of drivers alleged to have been involved in road traffic accidents;
- Terrorism Act 2000 – duty not to withhold information relating to the commission of acts of terrorism.

Therefore, you would be obliged not to keep this type of information confidential if questioned by the police.

Dealing with bullying and harassment

In caring and therapeutic environments there is an expectation that everyone will behave in an appropriate manner towards each other. However, from time to time, individuals and groups may develop behaviours that are viewed as bullying and harassment. This may take the form of nurses bullying and harassing other nurses or patients, or sometimes it can be the other way around with patients bullying or harassing other patients or nurses. In Chapter 1, it was highlighted that this was a feature of some of the institutional inquiries discussed. Bullying and harassment in any shape or form are not conducive to a caring and therapeutic environment and are therefore destructive. The Advisory, Conciliation and Arbitration Service (ACAS) is an organisation that offers impartial advice to employers and employees. It suggests that bullying is characterised by:

offensive, intimidating, malicious or insulting behaviour, an abuse or misuse of power through means that undermine, humiliate, denigrate or injure the recipient.
(2010, p1)

It describes harassment as:

unwanted conduct related to a relevant protected characteristic, which has the purpose or effect of violating an individual's dignity or creating an intimidating, hostile, degrading, humiliating or offensive environment for that individual.
(p2)

Box 7.1 contains examples from ACAS (2010) of some unacceptable behaviour in the workplace. However, it is difficult to give definitive examples in all situations as all behaviour is open to different interpretations by different people. Therefore, what is offensive, intimidating, malicious or insulting behaviour to one person may be found less so or not at all by another. People also make allowances for this type of behaviour depending on the context in which it takes place. For example, at some football matches swearing and shouting at opposing fans may be tolerated. In healthcare settings, staff may tolerate patients swearing at them if they are in pain or in the throes of psychotic episodes. In recent times the use of mobile phones and social network sites such as Facebook and Twitter has afforded people the opportunity to bully and harass others who are part of their social circle. Bullying and harassment can be part of everyday life for some people, particularly those with a learning disability, who often describe some criminal and abusive behaviour as bullying (Quarmby, 2008). See Chapter 4 (pages 73–4) on hate crime for more information; also, Mencap is so concerned that it has started a campaign called 'Don't stick it, stop it' (access the following page for more information: www.mencap.org.uk/campaigns/take-action/our-other-campaigns/dont-stick-it-stop-it).

Box 7.1: Examples of unacceptable behaviour in the working environment (ACAS, 2010, p2)

- Spreading malicious rumours, or insulting someone (particularly on the grounds of age, race, sex, disability, sexual orientation and religion or belief).
- Copying memos that are critical about someone to others who do not need to know.
- Ridiculing or demeaning someone – picking on the person or setting him or her up to fail.
- Unfair treatment, exclusion or victimisation.
- Overbearing supervision or other misuse of power or position.
- Unwelcome sexual advances – touching, standing too close, displaying offensive materials, asking for sexual favours, or making decisions on the basis of sexual advances being accepted or rejected.
- Making threats or comments about job security without foundation.
- Deliberately undermining a competent worker by overloading and constant criticism.
- Preventing individuals progressing by intentionally blocking promotion or training opportunities.

Activity 7.8   *Reflection and critical thinking*

Carefully consider the following scenarios and then answer the questions.

Scenario 1: During the afternoon staff team handover the ward manager holds up a can of deodorant, sprays it in the air and throws it at John Harris, an experienced staff nurse of 25 years. He tells him it is an early Christmas present from the team and Santa won't come to the ward unless he uses it every day. Most of the team had complained to the manager about John's BO problem and made jokes about it, but never when John was present.

Scenario 2: Stacey Napier is a third-year student nurse who has been asked to reflect, by her mentor, on providing health promotion advice to overweight patients when she herself is overweight and a smoker.

Scenario 3: David Kay, a gay community nurse, has recently moved teams and, on meeting his line manager for the first time, was told by him that he was too good looking to be a nurse and should have gone into modelling. His manager tells everyone in the team that there is a god as he has sent David to brighten up his life and add a little sparkle.

In terms of reflecting on each situation, answer the following questions.

- How would you feel and react if you were the person giving and receiving such comments?
- Do you think there are any issues regarding bullying or harassment?

continued . . .

• Would you have handled the situations the same or would you have done things differently? If so, how differently would you have handled them?

Answers will be provided in the following text.

Hopefully, in your reflections, you would be able to see that making such comments in scenarios 1 and 3 would be viewed as being unprofessional. The first situation highlights a very sensitive personal matter. Having poor personal hygiene can have an impact on those around you, both patients and colleagues. There may be an assumed personal hygiene problem with John or he might have a medical condition that causes him to sweat more or be sensitive to deodorants. The way the manager addressed the issue was absolutely the wrong way to go about it. If you were on the receiving end of this, in front of your colleagues, you would probably feel humiliated, insulted and very upset. If you examine the definitions of bullying and harassment, there are certainly elements of both, which gives John grounds for complaint. However, like trying to prove neglect, is it sufficient to look at this as a single event or does it need to be assessed over a period of time with a number of instances? This can be a debatable area, although it should be based on how the recipient feels. This matter could have been dealt with in a more sensitive way by the manager and, as a nurse, he should have been used to dealing with many sensitive issues. Picking the right moment, with the right person in the right environment may have had a more positive outcome. Remember to deal with such situations early and not to let staff make jokes about them behind people's backs. Caring environments and cultures should not allow this to happen.

Scenario 2 may have had a mixed response. Some people may have felt offended, while others may have felt that it was a legitimate issue to bring up. The key point here is that Stacey was not singled out for being overweight and a smoker. If this was the ethos of the therapeutic environment, everyone would need to be challenged regarding their own lifestyle in relation to giving advice to patients. Consideration may need to be given to other lifestyle choices such as drinking, exercise, diet and sexual preferences. If the team had signed up to this viewpoint, it would be difficult to utilise the bullying and harassment policy unless the manner in which it was pursued contained elements of this. Don't make snap judgements based on appearance and limited facts. Reflective practice affords people the opportunity to think about such issues at a deeper level.

Scenario 3 may also have had a mixed response. Some individuals may have felt uncomfortable about receiving such comments, while others may have welcomed the attention and felt good that others felt they were attractive. In the past, nursing did have an image that female nurses were fair game for sexual innuendo and lewd comments. They almost became sexualised objects of desire and fantasy. The problem here is that, if this is encouraged, it creates an environment whereby such comments become part of the unconscious and people make them without giving a second thought to the likely negative impact. Therefore, it should not be tolerated and encouraged. David should have made it clear to his manager at the first opportunity that the comments were unwelcome and had nothing to do with his capabilities as a nurse, and that he is not there to brighten up the manager's life. By sending out this clear signal David would probably have nipped the behaviour in the bud and, if not, he would have evidence that he tried to address it at the start. If David did nothing and smiled or tried to laugh it off, chances are that it would have escalated. If he felt offended, he should have reported the matter so as to prevent others from receiving such unwanted attention.

Supervision and reflective practice

Nursing by its very nature is a stressful profession and this is particularly true when dealing with vulnerable adults at risk of harm. Dealing with survivors and perpetrators of abuse can be very challenging, as difficult personalities and behaviours can put a strain on the most calm and measured individual. Therefore, support mechanisms and strategies need to be in place for practitioners to discuss their concerns, feelings and needs in an open and honest way. The NMC (2008b) supports the notion of clinical supervision as a means of supporting nurses and improving their practice. Bond and Holland provide a definition of clinical supervision as:

> *Regular, protected time for facilitated, in-depth reflection on complex issues influencing clinical practice. It aims to enable the supervisee to achieve, sustain and creatively develop a high quality of practice through the means of focused support and development. The supervisee reflects on the part she [sic] plays as an individual in the complexities of the events and the quality of practice.*
> (2010, p15)

Clinical supervision is facilitated by more experienced colleagues who have such expertise, and continues throughout a person's career.

Activity 7.9   *Critical thinking*

Carefully examine the above definition of clinical supervision provided by Bond and Holland (2010, p15) and answer the following questions.

- Can you identify the main elements of clinical supervision?
- How does it relate to safeguarding?
- Is there a difference between reflection and reflexivity?
- How does reflection/reflexivity fit into this type of supervision?
- Are there any other types of support for practitioners?

Answers will be provided in the following text.

The main elements of clinical supervision can be seen as providing an opportunity and time to discuss situations, dilemmas and feeling related to clinical practice. As healthcare becomes more complex, more thought needs to be given to clinical decision making. Clinical supervision is also an opportunity to gain support and insight from others on how you are doing in practice. Clinical supervision is well established in social work and psychology but has not always been given the priority it deserves in nursing. It must become part of established nursing practice, particularly in safeguarding. Critical decisions have to be made in complex cases, which, if they go wrong, may lead to clients being abused or not receiving the appropriate therapies. Practitioners also need support when they deal with the breadth of human emotion in the contexts in which abuse takes place.

As can be seen from the definition, reflective practice is an essential ingredient of clinical supervision. In this forum, an experienced practitioner/supervisor is on hand to facilitate the reflective process. Reflective practice may take different forms such as reflection and reflexivity. Both McKay et al. (2003) and Lipp (2004) argue that *reflection and reflexivity are inextricably intertwined*, but they all agree that there are crucial differences. Reflexivity is seen as having a greater intensity compared to reflection, and it is a more immediate and dynamic activity. It requires the practitioner to become more aware of his or her own as well as the patient's culture, ideology and politics. Reflection, however, usually involves thinking about something after the event. Reflexivity demands a more conscious approach, whereas reflection involves showing ourselves to ourselves. Quite simply, reflexivity is a deeper level of reflection and they both lie at different ends of a linear scale. During clinical supervision, both types of reflective practice may be necessary depending on the nature of the safeguarding issue or process. There are other forms of support such as peer support, mentoring, coaching, psychotherapy and counselling (Bond and Holland, 2010).

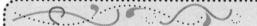

Chapter summary

This chapter has explored the meaning of the term 'profession' and how professions function. Professional codes of conduct and ethics can help both practitioners and the public. Practitioners are guided on how to behave and conduct themselves during their careers. A professional code may provide some help with ethical dilemmas. The public can gain reassurance that, when nurses fall short of expectations, there are a number of sanctions that can be applied to ensure patients are protected. There may be times when nurses may need to go public with their safeguarding concerns, but they should only do so as a last resort after going through a number of stages. Finally, nurses need to embrace clinical supervision as a means of support and improving their practice.

Activities: Brief outline answers

Activity 7.2 Reflection and critical thinking, page 129

The NMC *Code* (2008a) may be helpful with some ethical dilemmas as can be seen in Chapter 3. However, in some respects it may be rather limited in guiding nurses with their ethical dilemmas. Please read the following articles:

Pattison, S and Wainwright, P (2010) Is the 2008 NMC *Code* ethical? *Nursing Ethics*, 17(1): 9–18.

Tadd, V (1994) Professional codes: an exercise in tokenism? *Nursing Ethics*, 1(11): 15–23.

In terms of safeguarding, the *Code* is concerned with safeguarding throughout with both explicit and implicit statements. Explicitly, we can see this with the statement, *You must treat people as individuals and respect their dignity*. This clearly states that by doing this we should not be abusing patients/clients. Alternatively, the statement,

You must complete records as soon as possible after an event has occurred, indicates that by completing records as soon as possible we minimise the chances for mistakes to be made and the appropriate treatment to be provided, which implicitly means that we must safeguard patients/clients.

Activity 7.3 Reflection, page 132

Possible sanctions made by fitness to practise panels are:

- no further action;
- caution (one to five years);
- conditions of practice order (one to three years);
- suspension order (up to one year);
- striking-off order (no application for restoration to the register can be considered for five years).

Remember that, for the public to have confidence in a profession, there must be openness and transparency when it comes to disciplining its members. In the past, professions were accused of being too supportive of their members and acting like closed shops. There was a feeling that justice and fair play were not achieved and practitioners received minimal punishment. Often, the public and employers found it difficult to find information on nurses who had been found guilty of misconduct. Nurses and members of the public can attend hearings, as in the legal system, where they can witness at first hand how matters are dealt with and how both sides can argue their cases. This should ensure confidence that justice is seen to be done. It may be difficult for nurses to see their names and allegations against them put on public display, but this is no different from the current legal system and people have the opportunity to be found innocent, in which case this would also be there for all to see.

Further reading

Jenkins, R (2012) Using advocacy to safeguard older people with learning disabilities. *Nursing Older People*, 24(6): 31–6.

This article explains how advocacy may be used to safeguard vulnerable people.

Rolfe, G, Jasper, M and Freshwater, D (2011) *Critical Reflection in Practice: Generating knowledge for care*, 2nd edition. Basingstoke: Palgrave Macmillan.

This is a useful text if you want to gain a greater understanding of critical reflection related to practice.

Sutcliffe, H (2012) Understanding the NMC code of conduct: a student perspective. *Nursing Standard*, 25(52): 35–9.

This article was written by a student nurse who gives her understanding of the NMC *Code*.

Useful websites

www.acas.org.uk

The Advisory, Conciliation and Arbitration Service (ACAS) is a Crown non-departmental public body of the government that aims to improve industrial relations. It offers free impartial advice to both employees and employers.

www.pcaw.co.uk

The Public Concern at Work (PCaW) website offers advice on raising concerns in the workplace.

www.rcn.org.uk/raisingconcerns

This is the Royal College of Nursing (RCN) website for raising concerns in nursing.

Chapter 8
Interprofessional and interagency working

NMC Standards for Pre-registration Nursing Education

This chapter will address the following competencies:

Domain 1: Professional values

4. All nurses must work in partnership with service users, carers, families, groups, communities and organisations. They must manage risk, and promote health and wellbeing while aiming to empower choices that promote self-care and safety.

6. All nurses must understand the roles and responsibilities of other health and social care professionals, and seek to work with them collaboratively for the benefit of all who need care.

8. All nurses must practise independently, recognising the limits of their competence and knowledge. They must reflect on these limits and seek advice from, or refer to, other professionals where necessary.

Domain 4: Leadership, management and team working

6. All nurses must work independently as well as in teams. They must be able to take the lead in coordinating, delegating and supervising care safely, managing risk and remaining accountable for the care given.

7. All nurses must work effectively across professional and agency boundaries, actively involving and respecting others' contributions to integrated person-centred care. They must know when and how to communicate with and refer to other professionals and agencies in order to respect the choices of service users and others, promoting shared decision making, to deliver positive outcomes and to coordinate smooth, effective transition within and between services and agencies.

NMC Essential Skills Clusters

This chapter will address the following ESCs:

Cluster: Care, compassion and communication

1. As partners in the care process, people can trust a newly registered graduate nurse to provide collaborative care based on the highest standards, knowledge and competence.

continued . . .

Cluster: Organisational aspects of care

13. People can trust the newly registered graduate nurse to promote continuity when their care is to be transferred to another service or person.

14. People can trust the newly registered graduate nurse to be an autonomous and confident member of the multidisciplinary or multi-agency team and to inspire confidence in others.

Cluster: Medicines management

35. People can trust the newly registered graduate nurse to work as part of a team to offer holistic care and a range of treatment options of which medicines may form a part.

39. People can trust a newly registered graduate nurse to keep and maintain accurate records using information technology, where appropriate, within a multidisciplinary framework as a leader and as part of a team and in a variety of care settings including at home.

Chapter aims

After reading this chapter, you will be able to:

- explain the benefits for nurses working together with other professionals, particularly in relation to safeguarding vulnerable adults;
- identify some of the barriers that prevent professionals collaborating effectively in multidisciplinary teams and agencies;
- discuss ways in which interprofessional and interagency working may be improved to effectively safeguard vulnerable adults;
- discuss the implications for nursing practice of professionals and agencies working together.

Introduction

There are a number of potential gains for nurses in working with many different people, professionals and agencies in order to safeguard vulnerable adults. Health and social care are becoming far too complex for professionals such as nurses to work in isolation and be able to safeguard effectively the people they support and care for, so professionals and agencies will have to pool their skills and resources. This chapter will explore why we need to work together by critically reviewing the importance of interprofessional and interagency working in relation to safeguarding. Working together is not an easy task and a number of factors will be examined that may limit such an approach. These factors will concern issues such as professional roles and responsibilities, communication, information sharing, and team and agency dynamics. Consideration will also be given to exploring factors and approaches that may support better interprofessional and interagency working.

Coming together is a beginning.
Keeping together is progress.
Working together is success.
(Attributed to Henry Ford)

Interprofessional and interagency working

There is an increasing need for professionals and agencies to work together to provide services. This is due in part to increasing demand and complexity, and a need to use resources more effectively. It is also felt that a single professional group or agency would not be able to provide a range of services that complex cases require. Therefore, many government policies in areas such as learning disability (DH, 2009c), elder care (DH, 2001) and mental health (DH, 1999a) see working together as good practice in ensuring that clients' needs are met. D'Amour et al. (2005) also suggest that person-centred care is best achieved by a collaborative teamwork approach. However, there can be confusion around terms such as interprofessional, multiprofessional, multidisciplinary, interagency, collaboration, coordination and teamwork, which are often used interchangeably.

Activity 8.1   *Critical thinking*

Write down what you think each of the following terms means in practice and then identify differences and similarities:

- interprofessional working
- multiprofessional working
- interagency working
- collaboration
- coordination
- teamwork.

Once you have completed this, see if the NMC *Code* (2008a) supports nurses working with others and what specific guidance it offers.

Answers will be provided in the following text.

It is very difficult to find definitions of different types of team working as they are often out of tune with current understanding (McCallin, 2001). The use of such prefixes as inter- (between), multi- (many) and trans- (across) should give an indication of the type of professional working. Payne (2000) therefore suggests, on the one hand, that multiprofessional, multidisciplinary and multi-agency work indicate that there are a number of agencies and professionals whose skills and knowledge form part of a structure that provides services. They tend not to adapt their roles and functions, and not to cross professional boundaries. On the other hand, interprofessional, interdisciplinary and interagency working implies a willingness to cross agency and professional boundaries. Roles and responsibilities are adapted with skills and knowledge in order to meet service and client needs. However, these terms are used so randomly that they often do not reflect the true nature of professional working relationships in practice.

Payne (2000, p27) offers the following definitions:

- Coordination – *the need to achieve better relationships between the objectives and organisation of different agencies.*
- Collaboration – *people working together between different agencies and services to improve coordination in practice.*
- Teamwork – *collaboration between people in regular working relationships concerned with the same group of clients.*

Lawson (2004) argues that collaboration is a complex intervention with multiple components and has a number of potential benefits in areas such as efficiency, effectiveness, resources and social development. He feels that collaboration is a strong feature of competent practice, and failure to collaborate may be viewed as negligence and poor practice. Molyneux (2001) feels that the key to developing teams that work well together is to appoint experienced, motivated and committed staff who have a willingness to be flexible and adaptable. Confidence in their own professional role should allow for working across professional boundaries.

The NMC strongly supports the idea of working together as it includes the following statements to that effect in its *Code* (2008a) (see Box 8.1 for statements relating to working with colleagues).

Box 8.1: The NMC *Code* on working together (2008a, p5)

Work with others to protect and promote the health and wellbeing of those in your care, their families and carers, and the wider community

Share information with your colleagues

21. *You must keep your colleagues informed when you are sharing the care of others.*
22. *You must work with colleagues to monitor the quality of your work and maintain the safety of those in your care.*
23. *You must facilitate students and others to develop their competence.*

Work effectively as part of a team

24. *You must work cooperatively within teams and respect the skills, expertise and contributions of your colleagues.*
25. *You must be willing to share your skills and experience for the benefit of your colleagues.*
26. *You must consult and take advice from colleagues when appropriate.*
27. *You must treat your colleagues fairly and without discrimination.*
28. *You must make a referral to another practitioner when it is in the best interests of someone in your care.*

Not everyone agrees that interprofessional collaboration leads to improvements in care, as Schmitt (2001) questions whether there is sound evidence to support this view. In spite of this scepticism, research is beginning to emerge which shows that interdisciplinary working can lead to improvements in patient outcomes. For example, Saltvedt et al. (2002) found that the promotion of interdisciplinary assessments of older people reduced mortality rates by 50 per cent. More recently, Kesson et al. (2012) have suggested that breast cancer survival rates for women could be improved by the introduction of multidisciplinary team working in hospitals. In the UK, multidisciplinary teams provide the main framework in which multiprofessional care is delivered. This can, of course, involve both specialist and mainstream services working together to meet the needs of clients. There are distinct advantages put forward by Mathias and Thompson (2001) in adopting a multidisciplinary teamwork approach, which include:

- more efficient use of staff resources;
- specialists being encouraged to concentrate on the development of specialist skills;
- the facilitation of preventative work and service planning with an emphasis on holistic care.

Working together in the context of safeguarding

Tragically, there are many cases in which children have been abused and murdered at the hands of families and carers, and in which professionals have failed to share information. The inquiries into such cases as Maria Colwell in 1973, Victoria Climbié in 2000 and baby Peter in 2008 highlight poor working practices and communication between agencies and professionals. In some cases information may have been shared but the importance or relevance was not stressed enough or even picked up. It is not only in child safeguarding that these issues occur, but also in adult safeguarding, as can been seen in Box 8.2.

Box 8.2: Information sharing, Vale of Glamorgan Council, 2009

An 18-year-old man with learning disabilities was placed with a host family as part of an adult placement scheme. These schemes place vulnerable adults, such as those with learning disabilities, with host families who are carefully vetted and receive payment for the care given. This can be a very successful and cost-effective approach, and means that vulnerable adults are not always placed in residential care environments when they have nobody to care for them. The vulnerable adult in this case left children's services with a known history of disturbed sexual behaviour towards children. This information was not passed on by a social worker to the adult placement team, who then placed him in good faith with a family who had two young children. He later went on to sexually abuse both children. The abuser was later jailed and the social worker who failed to pass on information was later sacked and also removed from the register of social care workers. One of the positive outcomes of this tragic case is that now equal emphasis is placed on risk assessment of the vulnerable adult and the risks they may pose to potential host families as well as the risk others pose to the vulnerable adult.

(The BBC News report of this case can be accessed at http://news.bbc.co.uk/1/hi/wales/south_east/8055067.stm.)

The above case illustrates the crucial importance of sharing information, particularly during a transition period when a client moves from one agency to another. This situation was preventable but the catastrophic outcome will likely live with all those concerned for the rest of their lives. Ironically, social workers view information sharing as a particular strength of safeguarding in a multi-agency context (Pinkney et al., 2008). It is not just information sharing that needs to occur when working to safeguard vulnerable adults. The following case study illustrates the complexities involved.

Case study: George Thomas

George Thomas is a 54-year-old man with motor neurone disease (see Box 8.3), who lives with his wife and 16-year-old daughter and 22-year-old son. George is now totally dependent on his wife for all his needs and she is supported by a number of nurses who are supplied by the NHS. He has the use of an electric wheelchair and uses a communication aid to make his needs known. His son from a previous marriage has cerebral palsy and needs help with most daily living tasks, although he likes to do as much for himself as possible. He is able to talk but can only be understood by close family, friends and carers. He also has epilepsy, which is reasonably well controlled, although his infrequent seizures can be severe and life threatening, particularly when he is much stressed. George's wife is finding the situation very difficult, particularly as she is going through the menopause, and at times she tells George that she wishes he would hurry up and die. Their daughter was sexually abused by George's brother when she was 11 years old and is very withdrawn. George is anxious that his wife will not want to care for his son when he eventually dies as they have a strained relationship, although she understands his son's speech best of all.

Box 8.3: Motor neurone disease and cerebral palsy

Motor neurone disease (MND) is a rare and incurable neurological disease that causes damage to the nervous system leading to muscle damage and wasting. The specialist nerve cells particularly affected are those controlling speech, mobility, swallowing and breathing. The disease progresses until virtually total paralysis occurs and breathing becomes very difficult. Life expectancy, depending on the type of MND, is usually very poor, although some, such as the physicist Stephen Hawking, have survived for 40+ years since diagnosis.

Cerebral palsy (CP) is an umbrella term for a number of conditions that result in involuntary movement and/or a lack of coordination. There are often difficulties with perception, sensation, cognition, communication and behaviour. Some individuals may also have epilepsy and each person's CP will be unique; therefore, treatments and therapies are tailored to individual needs. Many individuals can lead relatively successful and independent lives if given the appropriate support and encouragement.

Access NHS Direct at www.nhs.uk/conditions/Motor-neurone-disease/Pages/Introduction. aspx for information on MND, and at www.nhs.uk/conditions/Cerebral-palsy/Pages/ Introduction.aspx for information on CP.

Activity 8.2 — *Critical thinking and reflection*

Consider the above case study regarding George Thomas and answer the following questions.

- What are the complexities of this case?
- In what ways is George vulnerable?
- What are the safeguarding issues for George?
- How would a multidisciplinary team approach be helpful in this situation?

Take time out to reflect on how you would feel if you were totally dependent on others. What sort of emotions would you feel and would you have a support network around you for support? As well as the websites mentioned in Box 8.3, access the MND website at www.mndassociation.org for some personal stories and information and www.scope.org.uk for further information on cerebral palsy.

Outline answers are given at the end of the chapter. There is also discussion in the following text.

There are a number of complexities concerning the case study that pose challenges to those charged with providing services as well as safeguarding. The first is that it is often not just an individual you are dealing with, but also the people who have a strong relationship with the individual concerned. This can be seen in George's case, with his wife and children and also extended family. It is the interrelationships between family members, good or bad, that need careful consideration and handling. Any proposed intervention would need to be carefully considered and planned as it may potentially be harmful to another person. For example, if George was suddenly moved into a care environment or hospice, this may be too stressful for his son, leading to a potentially fatal seizure.

In terms of George's vulnerability, this has been heightened with the development and progression of MND. He is now totally dependent on others for all his needs and, if they were not there to support him, he would not survive for very long. It is not just the physical effects of the disease that need to be taken into account; the psychological impact of losing the ability to do things and of dependency on others may have a even greater impact on the individual with MND. In spite of the gloomy picture, George's symptoms can be managed and his carers have a vital role in promoting a more positive attitude towards his disability in order to counter the negativity surrounding such conditions as MND.

The nature of the interrelationships between family members means that there are safeguarding issues for the whole family unit. Recent guidance by the Department of Health (2011a) regarding safeguarding adults suggests that safeguarding is developed by adopting six key principles (see Table 8.1 for how these can be applied to George's situation).

The final question in Activity 8.2 asks how a multidisciplinary team approach would be helpful in George's situation. The simple answer is that it is just too complex for one professional to deal

Principle	Example
Empowerment	George needs to feel in control of his life. People around him need to listen and act on his wishes and to offer encouragement and support in order to maintain George's sense of worth and control. All team members would be involved in the empowerment process.
Protection	Nursing staff need to closely monitor the relationships within the family, particularly the relationship between George and his wife.
Prevention	The multidisciplinary team needs to strengthen the relationship and bond between George's son and wife. They also need to enhance George's son's coping strategies in dealing with stress and future bereavement.
Proportionality	Risks taken should be proportionate to the potential benefits gained. For example, extra nursing support could be provided for George and his wife to go away on a break to strengthen their relationship. The risks would be that this may cause distress to his son and daughter. The risks and benefits need to be carefully considered and measured.
Partnerships	Links and referrals should be made with professionals to support the family unit. For example, specialist therapy and post-abuse counselling could be provided for George's daughter to deal with her withdrawn state. Specialist help could be provided for George's son with his communication (speech and language therapist), epilepsy (epilepsy nurse) and stress (psychologist or mental health nurse). A number of agencies and teams may be involved, such as mental health, practice and community nurses, and psychologists.
Accountability	All professionals involved in this case would be accountable for their actions in safeguarding George and his family.

Table 8.1 Safeguarding principles applied to the case study

with and it is not just George who may need safeguarding but other members of the family. Therefore, a multidisciplinary team approach would be essential in this case and you can identify particular professional involvement in Table 8.1.

Barriers that hinder professionals and agencies working together

---

Activity 8.3   *Critical thinking and reflection*

Read the case study below and answer the following questions.

- Why might Emily's exchange be helpful in improving interagency working.
- How might being based in a single building aid team working?
- How would the change in management of the team potentially impact on team dynamics and unity?
- What are the potential problems with a number of team members performing the same functions?
- What other known barriers exist that hinder professionals and agencies working together effectively?

Outline answers to the first four questions are given at the end of the chapter.

Case study: Emily Young

Emily Young has recently joined her local community learning disability team as a community mental health nurse. She is on a secondment from her community mental health team, which hopes the exchange will improve links between the two services. The learning disability team is currently made up of learning disability nurses, psychologists, speech and language therapists, social workers, occupational therapists and physiotherapists. They are based in the same building but each professional group tends to have a separate office. Emily keeps getting confused with the learning disability nurse as the other professionals think that nurses share a common training and have the same roles. Recently, the management structure of the team has changed and they are all now managed by a health team manager. In the past, each professional group was managed by a senior person who also provided professional advice. Emily is finding it difficult to fit in as she specialises in **cognitive behavioural therapy (CBT)**, *which is also undertaken by the psychologist and the social worker.*

There are numerous barriers that prevent professionals working effectively together in the best interests of the patients/clients they serve. First, there are differences in the understanding of terms such as teams and teamwork. A team is a group of people who come together, such as health professionals, and share a common purpose, while teamwork in healthcare is more to do with the process and actual performance in striving to meet set objectives. Therefore, disadvantages of multidisciplinary teamwork centre on the team as a working model and factors concerning ineffective teamwork. McCallin argues that *what is important is what teams do, how they do it [and] whether it improves patient outcomes* (2001, p423). Second, health professionals are seldom taught teamwork skills in which they work with other professionals and agencies (McCallin, 2001). Third, the lack of understanding of each other's roles, skills and knowledge base makes it difficult for professionals and agencies to work effectively together. Difficulties in teamwork can result when team members have a conflict in loyalty between the team and their profession.

Kvarnström's (2008) study also found that 'role boundary conflicts' had a negative impact on team dynamics as well as the knowledge and contributions of each professional, for example if a nurse started to undertake interventions and gave advice regarding posture and exercise, which are traditionally dealt with by physiotherapists. Tensions were also found to be raised when team members' views were not given equal status to those of other professionals or their views were ignored. Some of the other difficulties identified that hindered collaborative working were poor communication, not sharing information, some professions being given more status than others, organisational changes and a poor skill mix of professions (Kvarnström, 2008). The lack of team coordination, clear channels of communication, unequal work allocation and a failure to clarify team objectives can all lead to ineffective teamwork. There is also a danger that multidisciplinary teams may act as social control agents with increased power for the professionals.

Activity 8.4   *Reflection*

Imagine you are a student midwife in a multidisciplinary team in the following scenario. Would you feel you acted as a social control agent if you continued to promote breastfeeding?

Scenario: A young mother comes to you who wishes to stop breastfeeding her newborn child because it prevents her staying out late with her friends. She also tells you that she wants to get her figure back and her boyfriend is also pressuring her to give up. The team is very clear that breastfeeding is best, and some of the midwives and medical staff have put pressure on you to toe the party line and to continue to promote breastfeeding.

An outline answer is given at the end of the chapter.

There are similar issues with regard to multi-agency working. Atkinson et al.'s (2007) review of literature in this area found different types, models and definitions in operation, which made it difficult to make comparisons and evaluate outcomes. They also found similar barriers with regard to the difficulties of professionals working together, such as relationships, processes, resources, management and governance, communication and leadership issues. There was also a tendency for professionals' workloads to increase with multi-agency working (Atkinson et al., 2007). It is not just between other professionals that this problem occurs but also, surprisingly, between different fields of nursing. This can make it very difficult to safeguard individuals with complex needs.

Activity 8.5   *Reflection*

Try to identify the differences and similarities between adult, mental health, child and learning disabilities nursing in relation to safeguarding.

- Do we need these specialist areas or should we, like the rest of Europe, have a generic nursing programme?
- How would this impact on a nurse's safeguarding role?

Once you have reflected on nursing, try to identify the key areas of expertise of the following professionals:

- social worker
- psychologist
- psychiatrist
- occupational therapist
- dietician
- speech and language therapist
- physiotherapist.

Answers will be provided in the following text.

All fields of nursing share a common grounding in various aspects of nursing, such as life sciences, caring, clinical skills, handling and lifting, management, professional issues etc. In Table 8.2, the key areas of expertise are given for a number of professionals likely to be members of a multidisciplinary team. If you look at the expertise given for the learning disability nurse, other fields of nursing may lay claim to health assessment, promotion and person-centred care. However, each field of nursing obviously specialises in the areas of the client group it serves. The learning disability and mental health fields focus more on communication, values and beliefs. This is because many of the problems that people with learning disabilities and those with mental illness encounter are often caused by the negative perceptions of the general public. For example, individuals with schizophrenia are often feared because of their actions and verbalisations of their psychotic symptoms. In the previous chapter you would have read about people with learning disabilities being subjected to hate crime or indifference by healthcare professionals.

In terms of safeguarding, then, the common thread running through all fields is conformity with the NMC's *Code*, and now the latest *Standards for Pre-registration Nursing Education* and Essential Skills Clusters (NMC, 2010c). As has already been highlighted, everyone involved in health and social care should have a safeguarding role. However, the uniqueness of each field of nursing means that nurses from each of these areas have expertise, skills and knowledge that give them a distinct advantage when it comes to safeguarding. For example, if an individual with bipolar disorder was admitted to a ward with multiple bedsores and ulcers and was significantly underweight, a mental health nurse would be in a better position to assess whether this was due to self-neglect, carer abuse or poor management of his or her mental health condition. It would be unlikely that an adult nurse would have the level of expertise to make the right assessment.

Professional	Key areas of expertise
Social worker	Assessment of social care needs; developing, managing and evaluating packages of care; family therapy; provision of residential services/support; child/adult safeguarding issues; welfare benefits; approved social worker role.
Psychologist	Assessment of behaviour, development and social interaction; focused interventions (for example behavioural, cognitive, counselling); group work.
Psychiatrist	Assessment of mental health; diagnosis of mental health problems; prescription of medication and other therapies; forensic and legal matters.
Occupational therapist	Assessment of occupational, functional and interpersonal skills; assessment of the environment; provision of aids and adaptations; advice regarding housing design; provision of occupational and leisure opportunities.
Dietician	Assessment of nutritional needs; advice regarding healthy eating; health promotion; advice regarding special diets; provision of dietary supplements.
Speech and language therapist	Assessment of communication and feeding difficulties; enhancement of communication skills; developing communication systems; advice regarding feeding difficulties.
Physiotherapist	Assessment and analysis of movement; prevention of deformities and contractures; provision of aids and adaptations; advice regarding orthopaedic, respiratory and cardiac problems; advice regarding exercise.
Learning disability nurse	Promotion of a positive value base; person-centred care; assessment of health needs; health promotion; behavioural assessment and intervention; advice on and administration of medication; provision of residential services/support; development and coordination of care packages.

Table 8.2 Professional areas of expertise (adapted from Northway and Jenkins, 2007, p114)

Case study: Stephen Wilkins

Stephen Wilkins is a 44-year-old man with Asperger's syndrome (see Box 8.4) who currently lives at home with his parents and sister. He prefers to spend long periods in his room using his computer and watching violent and pornographic DVDs. His parents, both aged 82, are not in the best of health. His mother has angina and finds it difficult to manage the stairs and his father has suffered from depression for many years. In spite of these difficulties, his family is very close and supportive of one another. His older sister has taken over most of the caring in the house but suffers from panic attacks when venturing outside. She is severely overweight and has developed leg ulcers, diabetes and respiratory difficulties. She finds Stephen's behaviours problematic and only finds respite when she feeds him his favourite foods. David is Stephen's younger brother and lives locally. In the past, David has been very violent towards their parents when he has been low on money to support his heavy drinking and drug taking. His parents are frightened of him, but they will not report his threats and acts of violence to the police as they don't want him to go to prison. They generally suffer in silence and sometimes go without food as he has taken all their money. When David isn't drinking heavily he is very remorseful and helps the family by doing the shopping, cleaning, decorating, taking everyone out for trips, etc. He is particularly good at dealing with Stephen's aggressive behaviour and getting him to leave his room and go out.

Box 8.4: Asperger's syndrome

Asperger's syndrome (AS) is a type of **autistic spectrum** disorder that results in the individual having difficulties in social areas, such as interaction, communication and imagination. People with this syndrome have difficulties understanding some social norms and verbal and non-verbal expressions. AS is viewed as being on the higher end of the spectrum in that most individuals have average or above-average intelligence, but still have difficulties making sense of the world, processing information and relating to others. Some other conditions such as epilepsy, **attention deficit hyperactivity disorder (ADHD)** and **dyslexia** can coexist with the condition. The condition is lifelong and there is no cure, although people can learn to deal with their social difficulties. Many people with this condition can lead relatively successful lives with the right level of support and understanding.

For further information, access the National Autistic Society website at www.autism.org.uk.

Read the above case study concerning Stephen Wilkins and his family, and answer the following questions.

- What would be the special considerations in relation to safeguarding individuals with Asperger's syndrome?
- Which agencies or teams may be helpful to each family member?
- What are the particular problems concerning multi-agency working in safeguarding vulnerable adults in situations such as these?

Answers will be provided in the following text.

In terms of special considerations, it is important to view Stephen as a person first and not define him by his AS. As can be seen in Box 8.4, AS is a type of autistic spectrum disorder, which means that people with this syndrome have difficulties with the social aspects of life, interactions and communications that most of us take for granted. It is likely that Stephen will have some insight into his difficulties so may well be receptive to interventions that promote a more proactive approach to safeguarding. For example, his social and communication skills could be developed so that he would be able to read social situations better. He would also need interventions that help him reduce aggressive outbursts, and improve his general health and relationship with his sister. His brother, in spite of his own difficulties, may be able to help his sister in dealing with Stephen.

This situation again demonstrates complexity and the interrelationship between family members. Each member of the family has his or her own issues to contend with as well as relationships with others. There are a number of specialist agencies and teams involved with this family (see Figure 8.1). Stephen's parents would need the support of the older people's team for their health issues, which may include some mental health support. If this was not available, the generic mental health team may need to be involved as well for Stephen's father's depression. Stephen's brother would need support from his local drug and alcohol team for his addictions and the police would be involved with regard to his violent behaviour towards his parents. Finally, Stephen's sister would need support for her various physical and mental health issues, again from the mental health and community nursing teams.

As can be seen, a number of teams and agencies may become involved in Stephen's situation. A multi-agency approach was viewed as good practice and the best way forward in safeguarding vulnerable adults in the documents *No Secrets* (DH, 2000a) and *In Safe Hands* (NAfW, 2000). Both these documents gave the lead responsibility for adult protection coordination to local authorities. The reviews of both these documents (DH, 2009b; Magill et al., 2010) still support social care retaining the key leadership role with regard to multi-agency safeguarding at both local and national levels. There was also strong support for setting up Safeguarding Adults Boards (SABs), made up of a number of experts and an independent chairperson. However, in spite of the positive benefits of a multi-agency approach to safeguarding, there has been little research into this approach. Some research that has been carried out among local authorities and social workers has identified some perceived advantages, barriers and disadvantages in multi-agency safeguarding, although there are some conflicting viewpoints and findings reported (see Figure 8.2).

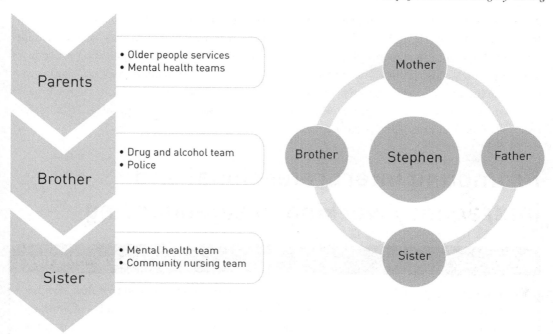

Figure 8.1 Possible agencies and teams involved in supporting Stephen and his family

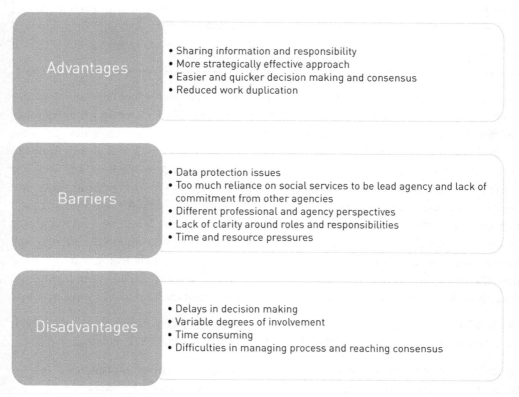

Figure 8.2 Advantages, barriers and disadvantages of multi-agency working and partnerships in safeguarding (Perkins et al., 2007; Pinkney et al., 2008)

A review of safeguarding arrangements within the NHS in Wales, undertaken by Healthcare Inspectorate Wales (HIW, 2010), raised concerns about health staff's awareness of vulnerability, safeguarding roles and responsibilities, and adherence to multi-agency safeguarding procedures. The Inspectorate also found a more worrying aspect in that some healthcare organisations were underplaying abuse as poor practice or as a complication of treatment. In spite of the areas of concern, good practice was highlighted in some areas such as responding to safeguarding issues, risk assessments in care plans and documentation.

Promoting interprofessional and interagency working in safeguarding

Activity 8.7   *Critical thinking and reflection*

Now that we have reached the final section of this chapter, you will need to reflect on what has been discussed so far, which has mainly focused on the reasons and benefits of working together and some of the factors that hinder this process. Once you have done this, think of ways in which interprofessional and interagency working can be promoted. Remember to be critical and also be creative in developing strategies. It would be helpful to revisit the case studies in this chapter, particularly that of Emily Young (Activity 8.3), which highlight some of the complexities and difficulties that need to be addressed.

Further information is given in the outline answer at the end of the chapter.

It is clear that, to effectively safeguard vulnerable adults, a multiprofessional and multi-agency approach to working must be promoted (DH, 2009b; Magill et al., 2010. However, we have already seen in this chapter that this is easier said than done. What is needed are common protocols, policies and systems, and clear lines of responsibility that all professionals and agencies need to sign up to. An important ingredient of working together is having a desire to do so, and also trust and confidence in the people you are working with. Negative attitudes built on mistrust, ignorance and working in isolation are a recipe for disaster. One of the first ways of understanding each other's roles, responsibilities and knowledge base and of building trust is to have joint training or education. In some European countries such as Finland, interprofessional education is well established, with social workers, nurses and other health professionals learning and mixing together at both pre-registration and post-registration levels. It has also already been highlighted that teamwork skills need to be taught and this would be the ideal environment in which to do so.

The RCN (2006) undertook a literature review of interprofessional education in primary care. It utilises a definition provided by Barr (2001), which states that interprofessional education is:

The application of principles of adult learning to interactive, group based learning, which relates collaborative learning to collaborative practice within a coherent rationale which is informed by understanding of interpersonal, group, organisational relations and processes of professionalisation.
(cited in RCN, 2006, p3)

The RCN distinguishes this from multiprofessional education, which it sees as just professionals learning together without the focus on collaborative practice. The key findings from the review were the need for a strong policy drive for interprofessional education and that most studies provided positive support for this approach. These centred on improving attitudes, knowledge and understanding of each professional role, patient outcomes and team-working practices. However, the review questioned the quality of most of the research undertaken into the actual effectiveness of this approach (RCN, 2006). Davies and Jenkins (2004) also raise concerns regarding the multi-agency approach to adult protection/safeguarding training. They feel that, although there are many positives to a multi-agency approach, such as that it encourages consistency and heightens the change of a collaborative approach to dealing with abuse cases, there is sadly little research that evaluates the quality of such an approach. They argue that such training may be watered down to such a degree that, although it may meet everyone's needs to a limited degree, it may leave some participants feeling less than satisfied. Finally, they argue that there is still a need for specialist training in safeguarding targeted at specific professional groups such as nursing (Davies and Jenkins, 2004).

Activity 8.8 — *Critical thinking*

- Building on the above points made by Davies and Jenkins (2004), what types of training in safeguarding would be suitable for a multi-agency approach? Also consider specific training for just nursing.
- Communities of practice are increasingly being used to improve practice by a number of professionals in health and social care environments. Find out more about this area of practice development and how such an approach may promote interprofessional and interagency working in safeguarding.

Answers will be provided in the following text.

Multi-agency training in safeguarding would be suitable for generalist areas such as awareness raising, types of abuse, legislation, reporting, risk assessment, health and safety, supportive strategies and service user perspectives. This type of education would also be suitable in exploring professional roles, working together, team building, communication and information sharing, and in developing positive attitudes to the multiprofessional and multi-agency approach to safeguarding. Generic training that spans all vulnerable groups and all staff types can never fully prepare nurses for an effective safeguarding role to maximum effect. Therefore, some specialist training for professions such as nursing is necessary. In the following case study, try to identify some specialist training needs.

Case study: June Rowland

June Rowland is a 59-year-old woman who has recently been diagnosed with fronto-temporal dementia. One of the symptoms of this type of dementia is that individuals lose some of their inhibitions due to the continued . . .

part of the brain affected. Her community mental health nurse has received numerous complaints from her husband and neighbours that June is making sexually suggestive comments and walking around naked in the garden. Her husband was recently arrested by the police for assaulting a man he found in bed with June.

(To find out more about dementia, visit the NHS Direct and Alzheimer's Society websites given at the end of the chapter.)

You may have found that specialist training should be around safeguarding a person with fronto-temporal dementia and working with families. This would be suitable for other professionals who may be involved in the case, such as a social worker or psychologist. However, cases of this type often raise specific issues for nursing, such as specific interventions concerning safeguarding, duty of care, adherence to the NMC *Code* and accountability. Phair and Heath (2010) propose a model for nurses to become involved in safeguarding investigations, which would require specific nursing knowledge and skills. This would be helpful with healthcare-focused investigations that look at health concerns, poor nursing practice, neglect and, of course, what appropriate nursing practice should be in place. The other consideration is that multiprofessional and multi-agency working may not be that well developed in particular parts of the country, so that nurses would have to adhere to specific 'nursing' policies and procedures.

In Activity 8.7 it was suggested that communities of practice may be helpful in a number of ways in improving professional practice. This may also be a useful way of promoting interprofessional and interagency working in safeguarding. Communities of practice have been used to evaluate interprofessional education (Lees and Meyer, 2011), strengthen education and practice partnerships (Berry, 2011), improve service in health and social care (Chandler and Fry, 2009) and finally improve the care of older people and the student nurse experience (Grealish et al., 2010). In the field of safeguarding vulnerable adults, this approach is less well developed. However, there are sorts of 'communities of practice' devoted to improving practice, such as the Practitioner Alliance for Safeguarding Adults (PASA UK) (see Useful websites in Chapter 4), which works in partnership with others engaged in the protection of vulnerable adults. You can see why they may be viewed as a community of practice when you see a definition of this approach. A community of practice has been described by Chandler and Fry as *a network of people who share a common interest in a specific area of knowledge or competence and are willing to work and learn together over a period of time to develop and share knowledge* (2009, p42). It is therefore easy to see why groups such as PASA UK may be viewed as communities of practice.

Berry (2011) draws on research to highlight some of the advantages and benefits of communities of practice that have been set up in healthcare. These centre on creating a sense of ownership, sharing resources and information, balancing individual and group learning, efficient use of time and breaking down cultural barriers across professions and agencies. A key requirement of such communities is the need for practitioners to engage in both individual and group reflective practice. In interprofessional teams, these communities have a skilled facilitator who helps to keep the group focused and effective. On occasions family members and service users/patients are invited to attend for particular issues and projects (Berry, 2011).

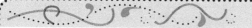

Chapter summary

This chapter has discussed the rationale for promoting interprofessional and interagency working as an effective way of safeguarding vulnerable adults. A number of case studies illustrated the complexities that professionals such as nurses have to deal with on a day-to-day basis. In actual and suspected abuse cases, the interrelationships between individuals require all professionals, services and agencies to work together. Nonetheless, a number of barriers exist that need to be overcome in order for this agenda to be moved along. The multi-agency approach to safeguarding is now well established in policies and procedures as well as in generalist training and education. However, there is still the need for specialist safeguarding training for particular professional groups such as nursing. Finally, communities of practice may offer further momentum for those professionals and agencies with an interest in improving safeguarding procedures and practice to learn and collaborate together.

Activities: Brief outline answers

Activity 8.2 Critical thinking and reflection, page 151

If you were to become totally dependent on others after a long period of independence, you would probably experience a range of emotions. The first may be shock or relief, particularly when you receive a diagnosis. Some people do feel relieved when they receive a definite diagnosis as they can often feel out of control not knowing why they are experiencing a range of symptoms. There may be an element of resentment: 'why me and not somebody else?' People may also feel anger at not be able to do things for themselves and being reliant on others. You may have been an impatient person in the past and having to wait for others to help you may be very annoying. However, it is not unknown for some people to actually gain some comfort and benefit from being dependent on others. Each person's experience and emotional response will be unique, so it would be difficult to over-generalise and have too much expectation that a person will respond in a particular way. You should find the many personal stories of people who have contributed to the MND website very moving and insightful.

Activity 8.3 Critical thinking and reflection, page 153

There is evidence that nurses do not work together as effectively as they should, particularly when dealing with individuals with complex needs, such as those with learning disabilities and mental health issues (Jenkins, 2009). People with learning disabilities are more susceptible to higher rates of mental health issues compared to the general population. Emily's exchange will hopefully break down barriers between the two services as long as there is a willingness from both sides to be open, honest and positive about improving links between different specialists and services.

The service being based in a single building should ensure that regular contact is made between different professionals, and should improve communication, understanding and trust (Atkinson et al., 2007). However, there is the potential that professionals may not mix as well if they stick to their professional areas or rooms, even though they are all housed in a single building.

Any change potentially can make people feel unsettled and lead to some resistance. Professionals may have genuine concerns about their lines of communication and accountability. They may feel that a manager who is not from their professional background may favour his or her own profession and not understand professional roles and responsibilities. However, although these may be real issues, it should be the leadership style and skills of the manager that are the prime concern. Tribal loyalties should be put aside in the interest of patients and clients as this should be the focus of developing effective services.

Undertaking extended roles and interventions traditionally performed by other professionals has always been a difficult issue to resolve. Working together will involve some blurring of roles. Each professional, due to his or her background training, will bring a unique perspective to performing different interventions. The key point here is that the person is competent to perform such a task or intervention. That is, has the person been properly assessed and judged by a recognised body to possess skills and knowledge to an acceptable standard? The NMC *Code* (2008a) is very clear that nurses should only work within the limits of their competence and base their practice on the best available evidence.

Activity 8.4 Reflection, page 154

In this scenario you may feel pressured to conform to the team's wishes and then exert pressure on the young woman. The important point here is that health professionals need to give information in a balanced manner and not make patients feel pressured into doing things against their beliefs and wishes. There is plenty of evidence to suggest that breastfeeding is best for young babies, but we cannot impose our beliefs on another, however much we would like to. We do not know the life situation of the person we are caring for, so having a night out without worry may be an effective strategy for her. Going out and having some freedom from caring may stop her from becoming anxious or depressed with her situation. It can be very difficult for a young student not to conform to the social pressure of the team and what we might feel society values.

Activity 8.7 Critical thinking and reflection, page 160

Some of the shared (multiprofessional) learning could be around finding out more about Asperger's syndrome, learning how to develop interventions, and improving knowledge and skills. Further topics on family dynamics, drug and alcohol abuse, older people care and safeguarding issues concern all of these three areas.

In terms of interprofessional education and learning, these would focus on collaborative skills development, which starts in pre-registration nursing education. This would involve being taught with other professionals, group processes and dynamics, working with others, dealing with conflict and assertiveness training. Placements with other professionals, teams and different agencies should help to break down barriers and foster collaborative practice. The use of secondments, sabbaticals and exchange programmes should help to place practitioners and students in a variety of learning opportunities in the UK and abroad.

It is important to gain patient and carer perspectives on multiprofessional and multi-agency working.

Further reading

Atkinson, M, Jones, M and Lamont, E (2007) *Multi-agency Working and its Implications for Practice: A review of the literature.* Reading: CfBT Education Trust. Available online at www.nfer.ac.uk/nfer/publications/MAD01/MAD01.pdf.

This is a very useful review of the literature regarding practice issues related to multi-agency working.

Davies, R and Jenkins, R (2004) Preventing abuse and protecting clients: a key role for the learning disability nurse. *Journal of Adult Protection*, 6(2): 31–41.

This article provides a number of challenges for learning disability nurses with regard to their role in safeguarding.

Goodman, B and Clemow, R (2010) *Nursing and Collaborative Practice.* Exeter: Learning Matters.

This text will add background and depth to collaborative working and care in nursing.

Phair, L and Heath, H (2010) Neglect of older people in formal care settings part one: new perspectives on definition and the nursing contribution to multiagency safeguarding work. *Journal of Adult Protection*, 12(3): 5–13.

This article offers a nursing role in a multi-agency approach to safeguarding older people.

Wenger, E (1998) *Communities of Practice.* Cambridge: Cambridge University Press.

This is an informative text and provides a framework for learning from communities of practice and how mutual engagement and development can be encouraged.

Useful websites

www.alzheimers.org.uk

The Alzheimer's Society is concerned with improving the lives of people with dementia.

www.eipen.org (if this doesn't work, try **www.swap.ac.uk/docs/projects/EIPEN2008flyer.pdf**)

The European Interprofessional Education Network is devoted to improving interprofessional education and multi-agency practice in health and social care in Europe.

www.nhs.uk/conditions/dementia/Pages/Introduction.aspx

This NHS Direct website offers information about dementia.

Chapter 9
A systems approach to safeguarding

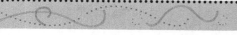

NMC Essential Skills Clusters

This chapter will address the following ESCs:

Cluster: Organisational aspects of care

11. People can trust the newly registered graduate nurse to safeguard children and adults from vulnerable situations and support and protect them from harm.

16. People can trust the newly registered graduate nurse to safely lead, co-ordinate and manage care.

18. People can trust a newly registered graduate nurse to enhance the safety of service users and identify and actively manage risk and uncertainty in relation to people, the environment, self and others.

Cluster: Infection prevention and control

26. People can trust the newly qualified nurse to act, in a variety of environments including the home care setting, to reduce risk when handling waste, including sharps, contaminated linen and when dealing with spillages of blood and other body fluids.

Chapter aims

After reading this chapter, you will be able to:

- identify a number of important components that make up an effective safeguarding system;
- explain how the components relate to each other and how the system should safeguard vulnerable adults;
- discuss how a systems approach to safeguarding may be applied to nursing practice.

Introduction

Safeguarding vulnerable adults has already been highlighted in this book as a complex activity that poses particular challenges to professionals, services and agencies. One way of addressing safeguarding issues is to have a number of approaches or systems in place. To be effective, these systems need to link together to form an overriding safeguarding system. A number of these key systems will be identified and put into context within this chapter. Specific attention will be given to exploring three such systems: clinical governance, risk management, and health and safety. The case studies and scenarios in the chapter demonstrate how such systems interconnect and ultimately fit into an overriding safeguarding system. Therefore, it is important to view safeguarding as a system of interconnected activities and roles. Sometimes, even when safeguarding systems are in place to identify vulnerable adults, it is reliant on professionals to act and when they fail to do so it can lead to tragic events, as can be seen in the headline in Box 9.1.

> **Box 9.1: Fiona Pilkington case: police face misconduct proceedings**
>
> In 2007, Fiona Pilkington killed herself and her daughter Francesca, who had learning disabilities, after years of torment from local youths. She and her neighbours, family and her MP had made numerous complaints to the police. A system was in place for dealing with vulnerable adults and linking incidents but this was not undertaken and acted upon. A number of police officers faced misconduct proceedings for their failure to safeguard the family.
>
> (See *The Guardian*, 24 May 2011 at www.guardian.co.uk/uk/2011/may/24/fiona-pilkington-police-misconduct-proceedings.)

What is a systems approach to safeguarding?

At any point in time we are all connected to some type of system. Most systems would be connected to other multiple systems. Indeed, our body is made up a number of systems that work in unison to keep us alive. Breakdowns in single or multiple systems can lead to illness or disease and, if it is fundamental, then death can occur. Systems are, therefore, collections of components, parts or structures that are interconnected for a common purpose. The key here is the common purpose that often defines the nature of that particular system. A systems approach would focus on a particular area, for example nursing practice, and would involve all the systems connected to that profession. Each system or component would affect others and requires coordination and a great deal of planning and organisation to ensure desired outcomes. A systems approach is nothing new to nursing as a number of nursing models are based on this principle. For example, both Neuman's (1995) and Johnson's (1990) systems models are based on systems interconnected with areas such as stress and behaviour. Even one of the most popular nursing models, from Roper et al. (1983), has a number of activities connected to aspects of daily living.

> **Activity 9.1**   *Critical thinking and reflection*
>
> • Consider how a systems approach might be applied to safeguarding.
> • Identify some components that might make up a safeguarding 'system' and how they might link to each other.
>
> *Answers will be provided in the following text.*

With regard to Activity 9.1, health and social care services require a systems approach in order to safeguard patients and clients. In a number of abuse inquiries, system failures have been identified as possible reasons for abuse occurring or going undetected for long periods of time.

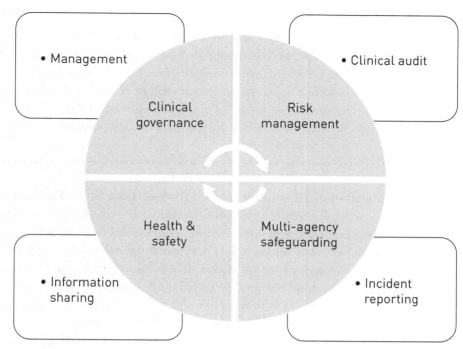

Figure 9.1 Safeguarding systems

For example, the recent Mid Staffordshire NHS Foundation Trust inquiry (Francis, 2010) found system failures in a number of areas such as nursing, risk management, clinical governance, incident reporting, information, management, infection control and audit systems. In Figure 9.1 you can see some of the key systems that may be involved in healthcare safeguarding. In the following sections of this chapter, health and safety, clinical governance and risk management will be discussed in more detail, with an emphasis on how these systems link together in order to safeguard vulnerable adults.

The importance of the other systems involved in safeguarding outside the inner circle shown in Figure 9.1, namely information sharing, clinical audit, incident reporting and management, can be seen in the following case study.

Case study: Halina Gorski

Halina Gorski is a 73-year-old Polish woman who speaks very little English and has recently been admitted to the respiratory ward of her local general hospital. The majority of the 30 patients on the ward are older people. Her daughter and sisters have been going in to visit her for a number of days, spending a large amount of time on the ward. Over a period of a week her daughter notices that her mother has had very little contact with the nursing staff and she has to keep asking for information regarding her mother's condition. At times, the nurses look very busy, but on other occasions they spend a great deal of time sitting around in the nurses' station laughing and joking. Her mother has eaten very little as she finds the food rather bland. The nurses

continued . . .

*have told the relatives to bring Polish food in for her if she hates the British diet. The lock on the bathroom is broken, so Halina is reluctant to use it and consequently smells quite strongly of urine. The **venflon** in her arm keeps sliding out and one of the nurses told her daughter it is easy to slide back in again and to just do it as they are very busy dealing with British patients without relatives. Halina's **nebuliser** has run out of medication on two occasions and the nurses took around two hours to deal with it. Halina does not want to cause a fuss and has asked her daughter and sisters not to complain because she is frightened of the nurses.*

It can be seen in this case study that there are a number of safeguarding issues. The first concerns the information and reporting systems. It is clear that the patient and relatives are not being kept informed of the planned programme of care. The information has to be sought by relatives rather than being provided at timely intervals. It is not clear if the information is provided in a language or form that can be understood by Halina. If she cannot understand what is being proposed or asked, she cannot consent or provide accurate information for her assessment and recovery. Second, the nursing staff seem to want to foster a view that, because they are short-staffed, it is all right for standards to slip. This is where an audit of standards of care is essential to ensure that good practice is established. In Figure 9.2 you can see a safeguarding practice circle. The main thrust of safeguarding should be to establish and promote good practice so that the segments of poor or abusive practice are reduced or eliminated and the whole circle just contains good practice. Abusive practice has no place in any practice circle. If patients feel frightened to report concerns, there is something very fundamentally wrong with the culture on the ward. A clinical audit should pick up these issues as well as those of poor communication, and environmental issues such as broken locks and the unappealing food.

Incident reporting systems are crucial to identifying and addressing potential poor and abusive practice. They should also be used to strengthen good practice and all three areas of practice in Figure 9.2 should be reported. Nurses are not very good at acknowledging that the basic care

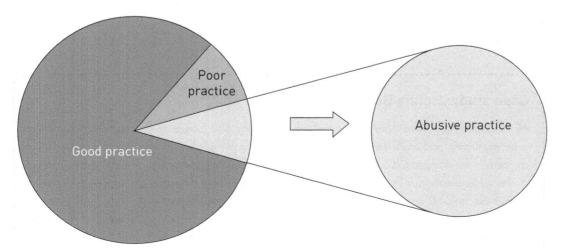

Figure 9.2 Safeguarding practice circle

they provide is valued by patients and the organisation (Jenkins, 2009). Patients' views should be collected as a matter of routine although, due to their vulnerability and dependence on nursing staff, patients may be reluctant to speak out or report bad or abusive practice. This is well known in healthcare so methods and approaches should be in place to overcome this issue. For example, confidential patient surveys cover a number of areas such as admission, general care, treatment plans, involvement, information, meals and overall satisfaction. These can be done while patients are on the ward or when they have left the hospital. As we live in a multicultural society a number of language options should be made available. It is important to make allowances for cultural variations. For example, in some cultures it is not unusual for family members to help out when a relative is in hospital, while in others it is. This also applies to cultural expectations of what should be provided by healthcare professionals.

The final system relates to management. In this case study, the management of this area is sadly left wanting. The nursing staff seem to be either very busy or idle, which demonstrates that care practice may not be being prioritised and systematised in an effective manner. The way care is organised needs to be seriously looked at, otherwise poor and abusive care will flourish. Some of the advice and comments made by the nursing staff are very concerning. Staff need to ensure that venflons are inserted correctly and made secure, and this should not be left to relatives to do. Potentially racist comments need to be addressed immediately as they often further alienate and disempower patients and relatives. There is a general lack of monitoring going on in this clinical area and this is a sure sign of a weak and ineffective management style. For example, Halina is having problems eating and the attitude is that relatives should sort this out. Poor nutritional intake while in residential care is a well-known problem for older people (Merrell et al., 2012) and as such should be given more priority than it appears to be in this case study. The omission of not dealing with such an important area as essential medication (Halina's nebuliser) is unforgivable and potentially may have had dire consequences. There is a general feeling of neglect within this clinical environment due in part to an apparent lack of leadership. An effective leadership style would have prevented this type of neglectful culture from developing.

Risk management

A key component of any safeguarding system would include risk management. Risk management is also a key component of clinical governance (DH, 2000b) and health and safety. The NHS Executive suggests that risk management:

> is mainly concerned with harnessing the information and expertise of individuals within the organisation and translating that with their help into positive action which will reduce loss of life, financial loss, loss of staff availability, loss of availability of buildings or equipment and loss of reputation.
> (1994, p1)

Risk management is therefore a proactive measure that utilises the expertise of its own staff to reduce the negative impact of a range of potential hazards and risks. These risks and hazards can potentially cause serious injury or loss of life. They can also leave a lasting legacy for an organisation with regard to its reputation (Box 9.2). The Corporate Manslaughter and Corporate

Homicide Act 2007 created a new offence of an organisation's gross failure in the way activities are managed or organised resulting in a person's death. Organisations can also face considerable penalties and individuals may be imprisoned as a result of their failings under health and safety legislation.

Box 9.2: Castlebeck

A number of care homes owned by Castlebeck, the company at the centre of allegations of abuse at Winterbourne View, have been closed (see Chapter 1, pages 12–13). Abuse of vulnerable adults at Winterbourne View in Bristol was exposed by the BBC *Panorama* programme in early 2011. The reputation of the company had been negatively affected as a result of the adverse publicity, which has contributed to the closure of some of these homes.

(See *BBC News*, 17 August 2011 at www.bbc.co.uk/news/uk-england-birmingham-1456 3038.)

Every member of staff has a role to play in risk management in alerting the organisation to potential risks and hazards that can lead to potential 'damage' to all parties (patients, carers, staff, organisation, etc.). Saunders (1998) states that risk management may be viewed at two levels, individual and organisational. At an individual level, risk management and assessment is undertaken as part of the care planning process. At an organisational level, service managers are responsible for identifying broad areas of risk within the organisation and instigating appropriate action.

Activity 9.2   *Critical thinking and reflection*

Carefully consider the following scenario and then answer the questions.

Scenario: You may have had a mild heart attack and your daughter has moved into your house to look after you. She will not let you lift a finger in terms of household duties – shopping, cleaning, cooking, etc. She feels you should take things easy and not exert yourself even though you have almost fully recovered after six months. You used to go out drinking with friends, have a smoke and place a bet in the local betting shop most weekends. She has put a stop to all this as it is too risky for you, especially as you fell ill in the betting shop. You now feel totally dependent on her and scared of falling ill again.

- What do you feel is the difference between a risk and a hazard?
- How would you feel if you were the father in the above scenario?
- Are there any safeguarding issues here?

Answers will be provided in the following text.

The answer to the first question in this activity can be found by reading the following Health and Safety Executive statement, which makes a clear distinction between a hazard and a risk:

- *[a] hazard is anything that may cause harm, such as chemicals, electricity, working from ladders, an open drawer etc.;*
- *[a] risk is the chance, high or low, that somebody could be harmed by these and other hazards, together with an indication of how serious the harm could be.*

(2011a, p2)

In terms of how you would feel in the situation in the scenario, we are sure some of you may feel you were in heaven, having someone to wait on you, hand, foot and finger! However, it is not possible to coast through life without encountering hazards and risks. Life is not risk free and there are a number of benefits to be gained from taking measured risks. Sadly, for many vulnerable and disabled people, taking appropriate risks has been denied them for fear of doing harm and not being in their best interests (DH, 2007). Essentially, they can suffer from being overprotected and 'wrapped up in cotton wool'. This can be seen in the above scenario, where the daughter is doing her best to protect her father from suffering another heart attack and possibly dying next time. She seems to believe that, if she cuts out all the risks, he will be safe from harm. However, in order for him to improve his health, he needs to take some risks.

Health here includes not only the physical but also the psychological and social aspects. We know that stopping smoking, increasing exercise and having a healthy diet is good for you. However, he could drink in moderation and have the occasional high-fat snack. For his psychological health he needs to have some control of his life as well as friendships and activities for his social health. Just because he fell ill in the betting shop does not mean this place is exceptionally risky. Obviously, any excessive gambling can potentially bring on other health problems such as anxiety and depression. This has to be balanced with the potential pleasure the individual gains from such activities. The safeguarding issue here is that, although the person has recovered from the initial heart attack, his dependence on his daughter and risk-free lifestyle has created fertile ground for the development of other health problems highlighted above. Therefore, it could be argued that his needs are being neglected and it is the sort of situation where he is being slowly 'abused' with kindness.

Activity 9.3   *Critical thinking and reflection*

Who do you imagine would have made the following comment?

Stupid risks are what makes life worth living. Now your mother, she's the steady type and that's fine in small doses, but me, I'm a risk taker. That's why I have so many adventures!

Now consider the following questions.

- In relation to the above comments, is this the type of philosophy that nurses should be following?
- What are your perceptions of risk taking? Is it a positive or negative activity?

continued . . .

- Make a list of terms used to describe both positive and negative aspects of risk taking.
- Do you feel it is important for vulnerable adults to take risks?

Answers will be provided in the following text. Additional information is given at the end of the chapter.

The above philosophy is rather carefree and 'stupid risks' will almost certainly have negative outcomes. Being able to determine one's own destiny in life is a fundamental human right and this was explored in Chapter 6. We all make decisions that sometimes pay off and sometimes don't. It is part of what we value as human beings, this freedom to control our lives. However, such decisions when we take risks, if they are not carefully thought through, can have dire consequences, for example crossing the road without looking or deciding to repair an electrical appliance without switching off the mains supply. There are always consequences to the decisions we make. It is often thought that vulnerable adults are not capable of taking sensible risks. Alaszewski and Alaszewski (2011) highlight that vulnerable people such as those with learning disabilities are aware of the everyday risks of life and are capable of learning from and managing such risks. They stress the importance of positive risk taking for the individual in increasing confidence, dignity and respect, as it would demonstrate normality. On the other side of the coin, risk-averse approaches have the potential to reinforce dependency, slow down development and deny vulnerable groups of people the opportunities to learn from experience. Fyson and Kitson (2010) highlight that the problem professionals face in working with people with learning disabilities is how to meet their needs in ways that simultaneously both safeguard and enable the vulnerable adult.

It is not only people with learning disabilities who have suffered as a result of risk-averse approaches. The Department of Health (2007) has issued guidance with regard to risk management in mental health services (see Box 9.3). It stresses the importance of positive risk taking; risk management should be mindful of how this can aid recovery and be part of an effective care plan. Explicitly and implicitly in this guidance are a number of safeguarding systems that can be helpful in the process. These include multi-agency and multidisciplinary teams, training and competence building, mental health legislation, partnerships, risk assessment and management, information sharing, health and safety, and management.

Box 9.3: Best practice points for effective risk management in mental health services (Adapted from DH, 2007, pp5–6)

Introduction
- Best practice involves making decisions based on knowledge of the research evidence, knowledge of the individual service user and their social context, knowledge of the service user's own experience, and clinical judgement.

Fundamentals

- Positive risk management as part of a carefully constructed plan is a required competence for all mental health practitioners.
- Risk management should be conducted in a spirit of collaboration and based on a relationship between the service user and his or her carers that is as trusting as possible.
- Risk management must be built on a recognition of the service user's strengths and should emphasise recovery.
- Risk management requires an organisational strategy as well as efforts by the individual practitioner.

Basic ideas in risk management

- Risk management involves developing flexible strategies aimed at preventing any negative event from occurring or, if this is not possible, minimising the harm caused.
- Risk management should take into account that risk can be both general and specific, and that good management can reduce and prevent harm.
- Knowledge and understanding of mental health legislation are important components of risk management.
- The risk management plan should include a summary of all risks identified, formulations of the situations in which identified risks may occur, and actions to be taken by practitioners and the service user in response to crisis.
- Where suitable tools are available, risk management should be based on assessment using the structured clinical judgement approach.
- Risk assessment is integral to deciding on the most appropriate level of risk management and the right kind of intervention for a service user.

Working with service users and carers

- All staff involved in risk management must be capable of demonstrating sensitivity and competence in relation to diversity in race, faith, age, gender, disability and sexual orientation.
- Risk management must always be based on awareness of the capacity for the service user's risk level to change over time, and a recognition that each service user requires a consistent and individualised approach.

Individual practice and team working

- Risk management plans should be developed by multidisciplinary and multi-agency teams operating in an open, democratic and transparent culture that embraces reflective practice.
- All staff involved in risk management should receive relevant training, which should be updated at least every three years.
- A risk management plan is only as good as the time and effort put into communicating its findings to others.

Carefully consider the following scenario and then answer the questions.

Scenario: You have to organise a day trip for two older people who wish to travel to a local derby football match. One has to use a wheelchair while the other, who is partially sighted, has a habit of wandering away.

- How would you go about undertaking a risk assessment?
- What are some of the main risks and benefits of going on this trip?
- How would you determine whether the risks would be worth taking?

Answers will be provided in the following text.

The questions posed in Activity 9.4 are about how we measure risks so that we promote positive risk taking. The answers to the questions can be answered by reading *Five Steps to Risk Assessment* (HSE, 2011a), which provides guidance on the five steps to take to reduce risks in the workplace (see Table 9.1). These steps should be followed in order to ensure risks are properly controlled and managed.

At some point in your decision-making process you need to carefully weigh up the potential hazards, and the likelihood of them happening, with the potential gains. In relation to the scenario, going to a football match should be a pleasurable experience and for most people this is the case. It is easy to see the potential gains in this activity for a vulnerable adult. This venture has the potential to be an empowering experience for the vulnerable adults (expressing choice, being facilitated to undertake the activity, normalising activity). However, there are potential hazards, such as football-related violence from some of the fans. The risk may be increased as this is a local derby, which has the potential to raise tensions between supporters. The other potential hazards would be the physical layout of the surrounding streets and of the stadium. Would the roads and stadium be suitably safe for wheelchair users? It would also be easy to lose someone in a large crowd, particularly if they liked to wander off. For the outing to proceed, the benefits should outweigh the potential hazards (see Figure 9.3).

Step	Action
1.	Identify the hazards.
2.	Decide who might be harmed and how.
3.	Evaluate the risks and decide on precautions.
4.	Record your findings and implement them.
5.	Review your risk assessment and update if necessary.

Table 9.1 Five steps to assessing risks in the workplace (HSE, 2011a, p2)

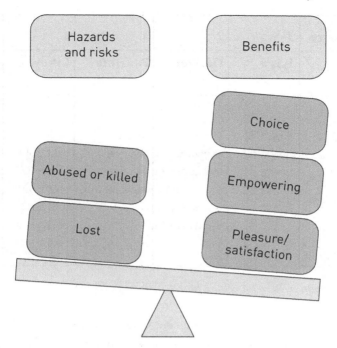

Figure 9.3 Potential hazards/risks balanced with benefits

In any risk-assessment process, once potential hazards have been identified the actual risk factor must be worked out. Remember the HSE (2011a) definition of risk highlighted earlier in this chapter, which stated that risk is the likelihood of it happening together with an indication of how serious it could be. To this end, the National Patient Safety Agency (2008) developed a risk matrix, which gives a measurement or scoring system of likelihood (see Table 9.2) and the possible consequences of risks (see Table 9.3). So, for example, if you were trying to estimate the risk for one of the clients with learning disabilities being crushed by a football crowd while in the stadium, you may score this 1 on likelihood, as it will probably never happen due to safety changes as a result of previous crushing incidents. It was always a very rare event. You also need to balance this with the potential consequences of the risk, which could range from minimal to catastrophic. Again, you may be able to use information from previous incidents for your assessment of risk. The risk of this potential hazard could be further minimised by careful planning and organisation of the trip. This would involve going to and leaving the stadium when there are fewer fans about (an hour before the game starts and an hour after it finishes), gaining support and knowledge from stadium safety officers and having an escape plan. Additional considerations in terms of calculating risk would concern the clients' ages, levels of disability, capacity, support needs, etc.

Clinical governance

Clinical governance was introduced into the health service as a key feature in which excellence in clinical care could flourish (DH, 1997, 1998, 1999b). Pridmore and Gammon (2007) argue

Likelihood score	1	2	3	4	5
Descriptor	**Rare**	**Unlikely**	**Possible**	**Likely**	**Almost certain**
Frequency: How often might it/does it happen?	This will probably never happen/ recur	Do not expect it to happen/ recur but it is possible it may do so	Might happen or recur occasionally	Will probably happen/ recur but it is not a persisting issue	Will undoubtedly happen/ recur, possibly frequently

Table 9.2 NPSA risk matrix: likelihood (2008, p8)

that clinical governance remains a strong influence in health policy in the UK and is an essential ingredient for safe, effective service delivery and professional practice. The influence of clinical governance seems to have remained, while some policies can fade away after a couple of years. Pridmore and Gammon (2007) do suggest, however, that there are differences in the application, interpretation and monitoring of clinical governance in the four countries that make up the UK. Remember that devolution will inevitably mean differences in policies and procedures in a number of areas. Clinical governance is defined by the Department of Health as *the structures, processes and culture needed to ensure that healthcare organisations – and all individuals within them – can assure the quality of the care they provide and are continuously seeking to improve it* (2011b). Currently, the Department (DH, 2011b) is developing guidance to help those responsible for clinical governance, such as clinicians, practitioners, team leaders and commissioners. Unfortunately, there is little evidence to suggest widespread uptake of clinical governance in the voluntary, independent and private sectors, although some do embrace this and other similar quality initiatives (Jenkins, 2009).

The Royal College of Nursing (2003b) highlights the particular contribution that nurses can make to this initiative, for example in areas such as planning services, consulting patients, team working, performance reviews and clinical audit. It also offers practical support and advice for nurses on how they can develop their skills and knowledge under the umbrella of clinical governance. Currie and Loftus-Hills (2002) argue that, while organisations may embrace the idea of clinical governance, it also needs to be seen by front-line staff as an integral part of their workload rather than as an optional extra of which they don't necessarily have to take too much notice. They suggest that there needs to be greater levels of partnership between clients, managers and staff if clinical governance is to be successfully implemented.

Domain	Negligible	Minor	Moderate	Major	Catastrophic
Impact on the safety of patients, staff or public (physical/psychological harm)	• Minimal injury requiring no/minimal intervention or treatment • No time off work • Increase in length of hospital stay by 1–3 days	• Minor injury or illness, requiring minor intervention • Requiring time off work for >3 days • Increase in length of hospital stay by 4–15 days • RIDDOR/agency reportable incident • An event which has an impact on a small number of patients	• Moderate injury requiring professional intervention • Requiring time off work for 4–14 days • Increase in length of hospital stay by >15 days • Mismanagement of patient care with long-term effects • An event which has an impact on a large number of patients	• Major injury leading to long-term incapacity/disability • Requiring time off work for >14 days	• Incident leading to death • Multiple permanent injuries or irreversible health effects

Table 9.3 NPSA risk matrix: consequences (2008, p13)

Activity 9.5   *Critical thinking*

- In what ways does clinical governance relate to safeguarding vulnerable adults?
- How does clinical governance in the NHS relate to a multi-agency approach to safeguarding?
- Discuss methods of making front-line staff such as nurses more aware of the importance of clinical governance, particularly as it relates to safeguarding.

Answers will be provided in the following text.

In terms of the first question in Activity 9.5, it has already been highlighted, in the earlier definition of clinical governance, that it is concerned with ensuring quality services and continually striving to improve care practices. Safeguarding is now more of a proactive approach in trying to empower individuals, improve practice and eliminate poor and abusive practice, and this should result in patients feeling safer. It is also easy to see why this fits nicely with clinical governance. With regard to the second question, it has been viewed by some that the NHS has largely taken care of safeguarding issues/incidents within its own clinical governance procedures with little regard to wider safeguarding interests (DH, 2009b; HIW, 2010). Social workers involved in safeguarding have felt frustrated by data-protection issues, NHS policies and procedures that hinder wider cooperation with, and reporting to, external agencies (Pinkney et al., 2008). This has led to the Department of Health (2010a) issuing guidance that links an adult safeguarding system within the NHS to the wider multi-agency collaborative approach to safeguarding. It has developed a flow chart on what to do when reporting safeguarding incidents (see the further reading at the end of this chapter). The hope is that there will now be greater openness and transparency regarding the reporting of clinical incidents to the wider safeguarding community. This should lead to greater partnership working and improved learning and responding to safeguarding issues by all those concerned with this area of practice.

Finally, Activity 9.5 asked you to think of methods of ensuring front-line workers such as nurses were made more aware of clinical governance as it relates to safeguarding. The obvious way is through both multi-agency and specialist nurse education and training. Nurses need to see how both approaches link together and also with the other systems that are involved in safeguarding. Serious case examples and reviews are good ways of demonstrating how everything links together. It has already been highlighted in Chapters 7 and 8 how clinical supervision, reflection and communities of practice can aid professional development. These are ideal opportunities to explore and stress the importance of clinical governance with the use of case studies and post-incident debriefings during individual and group supervision sessions.

Case study: Peter Adebayo

Peter Adebayo is a young man who is living with and cared for by his mother in a rundown inner-city area. He has recently been discharged back into the care of his mother from his local NHS psychiatric unit after a short spell of treatment for psychosis as well as drug and alcohol abuse. He was admitted after an overdose but is determined to stay clean. His mother has been showing signs of early-stage dementia but is fiercely independent and a devout Christian. Peter's community mental health nurse plans to visit him at home after concerns were raised by the local minister, who claims he caught a vomiting bug from the tea he drank at their home. He also claims that the flat stank of cannabis, with used needles lying on the floor and empty cans of cider. He said he was also shocked at the state of Peter's mother, who looked as if she had lost weight and had bruising on her arm. A day later, as he was walking past, the minister saw a number of people entering the flat with large amounts of alcohol.

Activity 9.6   *Critical thinking and reflection*

Consider the above case study and then answer the questions.

*   What are the safeguarding issues with this case?
*   How would such safeguarding issues relate to clinical governance?
*   What safeguarding systems need to be in place here?

Answers will be provided in the following text.

There are a number of safeguarding issues here. The first concerns Peter and a full assessment of his current mental health is necessary. This can be very difficult as drug and alcohol dependence makes accurate diagnosis of mental health status more difficult. This may also be a case of an 'unsafe' discharge as clearly his mother is having difficulties. There are obvious safeguarding issues with her and she would also require a mental health assessment. Their interdependence on each other needs careful consideration and, if either one's mental health deteriorates, that will have a considerable impact on the other. They are currently both potentially vulnerable to abuse. You do not know what events or incidents are taking place in the flat with groups of people who are drinking and possibly drug taking.

These safeguarding issues relate to clinical governance in that the responsibility of the local NHS Trust does not end when the patient is discharged. The after-care and discharge process needs to be investigated as the potential for harm is very real in this case. This would have dire consequences for the Trust if either Peter or both Peter and his mother came to serious harm. There are issues with infection control and it may be a case of educating Peter in the areas of food preparation and disposal of needles etc. Fyson and Kitson warn that *practitioners need to be aware that one person's freedom may be another person's abandonment to abuse and one person's safeguarding may be another person's restriction of freedom* (2010, p318). In this case, Peter was discharged into the presumed safe custody of his mother, thereby enjoying the freedom of community living. However, as the circumstances may have changed, his mother may now need safeguarding from Peter and his friends. If she were to be admitted to hospital this may well affect Peter's freedom. Remember, clinical governance is concerned with safeguarding and is about improving the quality of care.

In this case there needs to be much more monitoring in place so that the mother's health could have been picked up earlier. The systems involved would be multi-agency safeguarding, risk management, health and safety, reporting, multidisciplinary care teams and incident reporting.

Health and safety

An effective health and safety system at work is crucial in a safeguarding system. The Health and Safety at Work etc. Act 1974 is the primary piece of legislation covering work-related health and safety in the UK. It states an employer's responsibilities for health and safety at work as well as the employees'. A general duty of the employer is to provide systems of work that are, as far as is reasonably practicable, safe and without risks to health. Healthcare work carries many potential hazards and risks, for example catching infections off patients, needlestick injuries, working with radiation, surgery, contact with hazardous waste material, etc.

One of the main health and safety issues for healthcare professionals is harmful stress in work. Nursing is a particularly stressful profession due to the physical nature of caring and the psychological demands of dealing with complex and sometimes highly volatile situations (RCN, 2005). It can be like a roller-coaster ride, as one minute you are comforting a relative and the next you could be part of a crash team trying to save a life.

Activity 9.7   *Critical thinking and reflection*

Identify five common sources of stress in nursing. Then reflect on the following situations – how do you feel you would respond to each with regard to the potential stress it may cause you?

- Having to break bad news to a patient's relative.
- Trying to calm down a patient who is holding a knife.
- Helping a mother with the birth of her first child.
- Presenting at a conference to a large group of medical staff.
- Failing a student nurse for unsafe practice.

See the NHS Direct or HSE websites at the end of the chapter for further information on stress.

An answer will be provided in the following text.

McVicar (2003) undertook a literature review regarding workplace stress in nursing. He identified some sources of stress that had a negative impact on work satisfaction (see Figure 9.4).

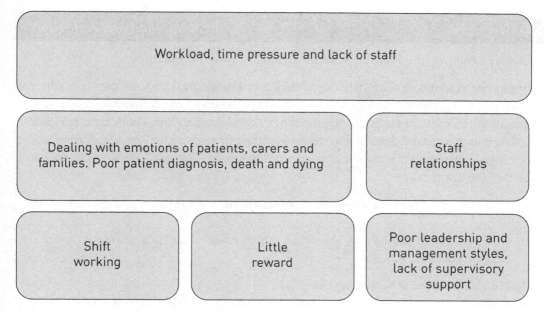

Figure 9.4 Sources of stress in nursing (McVicar, 2003)

As can be seen in Figure 9.4 there is a range of potential stressors in nursing. Each person may relate to a particular source as the one that causes him or her personally the greatest amount of stress. Workload, time pressures and lack of staff usually rank very highly with most nurses. Your responses to the various situations in Activity 9.7 will have demonstrated the individual nature of stress. Some people may relish dealing with the pressures illustrated in each of the situations, while others may have feelings of dread, anxiety, depression and other negative emotions. Sometimes you may feel you can cope with a situation but, when things change, you may panic or freeze on the spot. For example, assisting with childbirth is usually a heart-warming moment, but if the mother develops complications and the baby is stillborn your coping strategy may need to change. Skills, knowledge and competence (a key feature of this book) should provide you with confidence to master and cope with all of the above situations. However, it is also your self-concept and perceptions of the situations that are often the key determinants of whether you can manage the pressure or not.

To recap, stress can be positive as it may act as a motivator and keep you focused. The problem is with harmful stress. This is when the demands outweigh your resources to cope with the pressure. This is when the pressure begins to affect you physically and psychologically to the extent that it impacts negatively on your body, work and home life.

Activity 9.8   *Critical thinking and reflection*

Consider carefully the following scenario and then answer the questions.

Scenario: A friend of yours, whom you introduced to the local rehabilitation unit where you work, volunteered to transport vulnerable young adults to appointments and activities. You used to get them ready for these outings and chatted to him about their personal progress and problems. After a year the police arrest your friend for sexually abusing four of the patients, most of whom have poor communication skills, and one of whom he has made pregnant.

- What are the potential stressors in safeguarding vulnerable people in the above scenario?
- How can organisations and individual nurses ensure that they do not experience harmful effects of stress?

Answers will be provided in the following text.

All the stressors identified previously in nursing will apply as this is the context in which nurses work. However, safeguarding can pose particular sources of stress as can be seen in the above scenario. Here you may feel awful as you introduced the abuser to the unit and unknowingly provided him with important information he could use in order to abuse his victims. Your colleagues should be supportive and see that this abuser used his friendship to gain access to vulnerable adults. However, some may take an alternative viewpoint and point the finger of blame towards you. The relatives of the victims are more likely to do this as they will want answers and we are currently in a 'blame' culture. In Chapter 1 (page 20), it was highlighted that the proactive abuser actively seeks out potential victims and creates opportunities in order to abuse (Davies et al., 2011). You may have to deal with the process of adult-protection procedures and police investigations, such as making statements, and attending court and panel hearings etc. Then there is the issue of dealing with the abused and their relatives, and trying to come to terms with it all. The sources of stress may seem endless and lifelong.

In the following case study, you can see elements of the reactive type of abuser (Davies et al., 2011) (see also Chapter 1, pages 19–20), who abuses because of the stress he or she is under and this is often linked to a critical incident where the abuser finally 'snaps'.

Case study: Inga Schmidt

Inga Schmidt is a hard-working and highly thought of staff nurse who works in a very busy ward environment. She has to induct most of the agency staff working in this environment, which has a high turnover of staff due to a number of factors, such as the demanding nature of the patients, poor medical support and a lack of resources such as reliable equipment. Mrs Elizabeth Lewis, a rather obese woman on

continued . . .

oxygen therapy after a lifetime of smoking, is particularly challenging to nursing staff, often setting off her alarm for assistance for the most trivial reasons and making constant complaints. She often refers to Inga as the 'Nazi' to the other patients and staff but never within earshot of Inga. However, she saves her most savage verbal abuse for her dutiful husband, who just sits by her bed and accepts her tirades and physical assaults. Inga has been feeling the stress lately on the ward with an increased workload and shortage of staff. She has a son with cystic fibrosis and her mother is very ill in Germany. One day, after Mrs Lewis gives her husband a particularly nasty savaging and he leaves, Inga cracks and gives the woman a piece of her mind. She screams at Elizabeth that she is a nasty 'bitch' and then tells her that if she really was a Nazi she would take her out and shoot her. Inga also tells Elizabeth that, if she did not eat and smoke so much, she would not be in here wasting precious nursing time and taxpayers' money.

In this case study you can see that a normally efficient, hard-working and effective nurse has fallen foul of the pressures of work and her home life. Verbally abusing a patient in such a way, in just a moment, may put an end to her career as a nurse. The impact on the patient may be equally devastating, and have a negative impact on her recovery. However much the provocation, and in this case there was a great deal, it does not justify the actions of this nurse. This case illustrates the potential of stress to turn the 'good' nurse into an abuser.

There are two sets of responsibilities under which stress at work can be managed. The main responsibility for harmful stress reduction should lie with the employer, who should ensure that there is a safe system of work in place by managing stress effectively. The HSE (2011b) believes that this is possible by addressing six key areas (see Table 9.4).

Area of responsibility	Example
Demands	Workload, work patterns and the work environment.
Control	Amount of control and say in how employees do their work.
Support	Encouragement, sponsorship and resources provided by the organisation, line management and colleagues.
Relationships	Promoting and encouraging positive working relationships. Reducing conflict and dealing with unacceptable behaviour.
Roles	Role clarity and reducing/eliminating role conflict within the organisation.
Change	How organisational change is managed and communicated in the organisation.

Table 9.4 Management standards for work-related stress (HSE, 2007, p12)

It must be remembered that an overly stressed nurse is a potential abuser. Individual nurses as employees have a responsibility in managing their own stress in relation to the six areas in Table 9.4. In addition to these they can keep themselves fit and healthy and develop effective coping skills. It is a good idea to question and learn from staff who demonstrate this skill. Such individuals will often show assertive skills and provide an air of being in control. The use of clinical supervision and reflection can also help in this area by providing the context in which to learn. Nurses need to feel confident in performing a safeguarding role and this should come with having the appropriate knowledge, skills and attitudes (Davies and Jenkins, 2004).

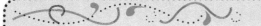

Chapter summary

This chapter has been concerned with how a systems approach can be used to safeguard vulnerable people. A safeguarding system comprises a number of other systems such as risk management, clinical governance and health and safety. These in turn are each connected to other systems with both different and similar functions. The effectiveness of a safeguarding system is determined by how well it safeguards vulnerable adults. In too many cases, abuse has been allowed to flourish due to system failures, particularly in areas such as incident reporting, information sharing and multi-agency working. Excessive stress at work can also put too much pressure on staff, leading to poor and abusive care. A safeguarding system is only as strong as its weakest link.

Activities: Brief outline answers

Activity 9.3 Critical thinking and reflection, pages 173–4

It was Homer Simpson (Episode 5F17, original airdate 5 October 1998) who said *stupid risks are what makes life worth living*, etc. Homer is a well-known character from the cult cartoon family, *The Simpsons*. He can be a reckless risk taker who often acts on impulse without thinking of the consequences of his actions.

The following is a list of possible negative and positive perceptions of risk taking.

Negative	**Positive**
Harm	Empowering
Dangerous	Dignity
Loss	Respect
Damage	Challenge
Unsafe	Learning new skills
Death	Opportunity

Further reading

Commission on Dignity in Care for Older People (2012) *Delivering Dignity: Securing dignity in care for older people in hospitals and care homes.* London: NHS Confederation, Local Government Association and Age UK.

Copies of this report are available via the NHS Confederation at www.nhsconfed.org/dignity, Age UK at www.ageuk.org.uk and from the Local Government Association www.local.gov.uk.

Department of Health (DH) (2010a) *Clinical Governance and Adult Safeguarding: An integrated process.* London: Department of Health.

This guidance spells out with the use of a flow chart what to do in terms of linking in to the multi-agency approach to safeguarding. The guidance provides two case examples demonstrating the use of the guidance.

Health and Safety Executive (HSE) (2007) *Managing the Causes of Work-related Stress: A step-by-step approach using the management standards*, 2nd edition. London: The Stationery Office. Available online at www.hse.gov.uk/pubns/priced/hsg218.pdf.

This text provides advice and guidance on how to manage work-related stress from identification to practical solutions.

Royal College of Nursing (RCN) (2003) *Clinical Governance: An RCN resource guide.* London: Royal College of Nursing.

This is a useful resource guide for nurses on aspects of clinical governance.

Useful websites

www.hse.gov.uk

The Health and Safety Executive is an independent regulator and watchdog devoted to reducing death, illness and injury in the workplace. It offers up-to-date guidance and advice to both employers and employees with regard to UK health and safety in the workplace.

www.nhs.uk/Conditions/stress-anxiety-depression/Pages/workplace-stress.aspx

This website offers NHS guidance on workplace stress.

www.npsa.nhs.uk

The National Patient Safety Agency aims to reduce risk and improve the safety of patients receiving care from the NHS. It provides up-to-date information and guidance on reducing risks to patients by improving practice.

Chapter 10
Safeguarding and research

Introduction

Activity 10.1   *Evidence-based practice and research*

Before reading through this chapter take a few minutes to think about why research concerning safeguarding is important.

- What aspects of safeguarding do you feel need to be researched?
- Why is such research important for the development of nursing practice based on the best possible evidence?

Outline answers are given at the end of the chapter.

Why have we included a chapter about research in this book when there are many research textbooks available? The answer is quite simple: we believe that research and practice should be considered together. This is true in all areas of practice, but especially so in relation to safeguarding, where we need to ensure that we are providing the most effective support we can.

Safeguarding adults is a relatively recent area of concern and this means that research in this area is limited. However, in Activity 10.1 you will have identified some reasons why it is important for more research in this area to be undertaken. This chapter is going to discuss the importance of evidence-based practice and examine some existing evidence. The challenges in undertaking research in this area will then be explored, before suggestions for possible further research are put forward.

Evidence-based practice

The NMC *Code* (2008a) requires all nurses to base their practice on the best available evidence or best practice. Evidence in this context includes research or other information that helps us to know what works best in specific situations, for certain groups of people, and for particular costs. It can also include research that helps us understand things, such as why certain things happen, how people feel about them, and what impact things have on them. Of course, sometimes research is not available, and in such circumstances it is necessary to use other information such as policy documents, official reports and respected opinions to inform practice. It is also important to remember that 'evidence' is only one element that has to be considered, as professional judgement and patient preferences are also important (Aveyard and Sharp, 2009). Even if the evidence suggests that a particular intervention would be most effective in a particular situation, professional judgement may tell you that, with a specific patient, it would not be the best approach, or it may not be acceptable to the patient. For example, the patient concerned may have an allergy to a particular treatment or may have religious objections to receiving it. Here, an alternative approach would be required, but it would be important to provide a rationale as to why this is the case.

In practice, there are many reasons as to why the best available evidence is not always used. Sometimes the amount of evidence is limited, practitioners are unaware of the evidence, or there are barriers to using the evidence in the practice setting. It is not possible here to provide a detailed discussion of evidence-based practice, and you might like to follow up some of the suggestions for further reading at the end of this chapter. However, it is important to understand the key stages of evidence-based practice so that you can consider its importance to safeguarding. Figure 10.1 sets out these stages.

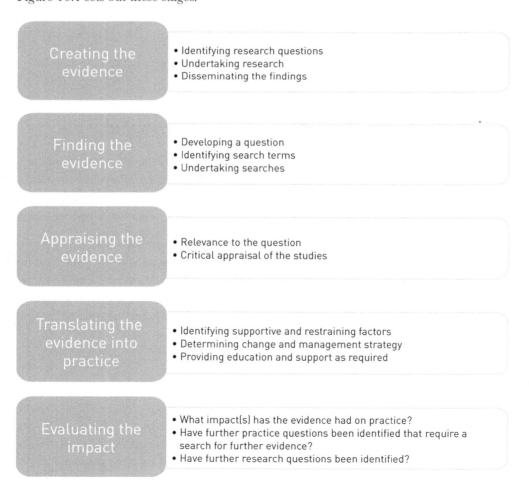

Figure 10.1 The stages of evidence-based practice

The first stage in Figure 10.1 shows that it is important that research is not only undertaken, but that its findings are also made available to others. If we are faced with a practice-based question, and we want to find the best available evidence, we need to be able to clearly identify the question, to identify the best search terms, and use these to search the most appropriate databases. To try this process complete Activity 10.2 before reading on.

Activity 10.2   *Evidence-based practice and research*

- Think of a practice question concerning safeguarding that you would like to answer. If you cannot think of a question at the moment, use this one: 'What is the role of the nurse in safeguarding older adults from physical abuse?'
- Develop a search strategy that includes the terms you are going to use to undertake your search and the databases you will use, then try undertaking the search.
- How many papers did you find? Did your search result in material that was relevant to your topic or did you find a lot of irrelevant papers? Were some databases more useful than others?

Advice on this activity is provided at the end of the chapter.

Having found some possible sources of evidence, however, you now need to assess both its relevance to your question and its quality. The first of these two assessments requires that you have clear *inclusion* and *exclusion criteria*. This means that you have to develop two lists of criteria that you will use to decide whether or not a paper you have found is relevant to your question. The inclusion criteria are those characteristics that each paper must have if you are to include it in the evidence you are reviewing. For example, if you were looking for evidence relating to the role of the nurse working with older people in acute hospitals, to be included the papers would have to refer to nurses working with this particular group in the specific setting of the acute hospital. The exclusion criteria are those that, if a particular study had them, would mean that it would not be included. Using the same example, an exclusion criterion would be papers that relate to nurses working with other client groups in acute hospital settings and those that relate to nurses working with older people in community settings. Using these criteria will mean that the number of papers you are left with will be fewer than those you started with. However, even if the papers are relevant, it is still important to review each of them carefully to assess their quality: it is important that we do not base practice on weak evidence, or evidence that is questionable due to the methods used. Please see the further reading at the end of the chapter for some suggestions regarding critical appraisal of research.

Having identified suitable research, or other evidence, the challenge is then to think about how best to introduce it to practice. This requires the use of other skills such as change management, and a useful starting point is to consider what factors you feel would support the change and also those you feel might work against (or restrain) the change.

Activity 10.3   *Critical thinking*

Imagine you are a newly qualified staff nurse who has been asked to take the lead on introducing some new evidence-based guidelines concerning safeguarding. What do you think might be the factors that might help you in implementing this change and what barriers might you encounter? Try to consider both human and non-human factors.

As this activity concerns your own ideas, there is no outline answer at the end of the chapter.

Having identified factors that are supportive of change and those that might work against change, it is then important to see how best to increase the supportive factors and, possibly, reduce the limiting or restraining factors. A clear change management strategy is needed and there are many of these to choose from (see the further reading at the end of the chapter). Change is often managed very badly or not managed at all: given the effects of not providing best practice in relation to safeguarding, this is something we must aim to get right. It is also important to understand that, having made one change, this may highlight the need for other changes and, as knowledge is expanding all the time, we should be aware of new developments and their implications for practice. While Figure 10.1 shows a process that seems to lead to an end point, the final stage should not be forgotten. All changes need to be evaluated and this may mean a return to the first stage of identifying further questions and evidence. So the process starts again.

Evidence relating to safeguarding

It has already been suggested in this chapter that research specifically concerning safeguarding and nursing is limited. This may be for a number of reasons, such as the fact that it was only in the early 2000s that we started to have policy guidance in this area and the term 'safeguarding' is even more recent. However, we have known for many years that abuse and neglect occur within the health service (see Chapter 1). This evidence takes the form of enquiries into situations where abuse has occurred, rather than research into the effectiveness or otherwise of interventions. Nonetheless, the reports indicate the presence of a problem, and suggest some possible factors that need to be changed in order to ensure that similar situations do not arise in the future. Despite this history (as was seen in Chapter 8), safeguarding has not always been seen as a key responsibility of the health service. This may be another reason why nursing research in this area is limited.

This limited amount of research specific to nursing and safeguarding means that, in order to provide care based on the best available evidence (NMC, 2008a), we need to be aware of what research does exist, and also to consider the relevance of research in two related areas:

*   research that has been undertaken regarding safeguarding in other settings;
*   nursing research that is not specifically related to safeguarding but that has relevance to this aspect of care.

To help you to think about these two areas, take time to complete Activity 10.4.

Activity 10.4   *Critical thinking*

Think about the two areas of research suggested above and try to identify possible topics of research that may be relevant. Try to think as broadly as you can.

Suggestions are provided at the end of the chapter and in the discussion below.

It may be relevant to consider studies undertaken within other professional groups such as social workers or counsellors. For example, McDonald (2010) examined how social workers use the Mental Capacity Act 2005 to make decisions where older people lack the capacity to make their own decisions. She found that different teams, and sometimes even social workers within the same team, made decisions in different ways. McDonald's findings may have relevance to nursing practice and help us to better understand how decisions might be made, since we also operate within the provisions of the Mental Capacity Act 2005. Another study (including both nurses and social care staff) examined the implementation of adult-protection policies in services for people with learning disabilities (Northway et al., 2007). It was found that, while policies existed, knowledge about them varied and challenges in practice remained. In relation to nursing practice, this suggests the need for close attention to be paid to policy implementation if safeguarding policies are to be effective.

Other research has relevance to safeguarding. For example, in the Czech Republic Buzgova and Ivanova (2011) examined violation of ethical principles and abuse in residential homes for older people. Data were gathered from 454 employees and 488 clients from 12 residential homes. The responses (particularly those from the employees) revealed both physical and psychological abuse. The older people who were most at risk of being abused were those who had dementia and those who voiced dissatisfaction. The staff most likely to be abusers were those who had been employed in residential care for over five years, who lacked adequate knowledge regarding social services and who suffered from burnout. While this study was undertaken in a particular care setting and in a different country, it is possible to see how its findings may be relevant to the nursing care we deliver. For example, if we are to safeguard older people, it is important that we understand who may be at greatest risk and also that we are alert to warning signs that may be displayed by staff. It also suggests possible strategies we can use to prevent abuse, such as ensuring that staff have adequate knowledge and that staff-support mechanisms are in place to prevent burnout.

Some nursing research has been undertaken that has direct relevance to safeguarding. For example, Lo et al. (2009) investigated how student nurses perceive and understand elder abuse. Their findings suggested that students did not feel sufficiently knowledgeable to fulfil the role expected of them on qualifying, in relation to identifying and addressing the abuse of older people. Sandmoe and Kirkevold (2010) examined issues relating to the abuse of older people, but they explored how community nurses in Norway undertake assessments in relation to suspected abuse. They identified that such assessments are dependent upon a range of factors that relate to the nurses, the clients, the specific situation and the community care organisation. The need to develop a framework to facilitate assessment in this context is proposed. Winterstein (2012) continues the theme of nursing, and elder abuse and neglect, by undertaking interviews with experienced nurses in Israel. The need to raise awareness regarding elder abuse, and the importance of training that allows issues such as ethical concerns to be raised and discussed, are noted.

When considering the evidence base relating to safeguarding, it is also important to think carefully about the various dimensions that may be of interest, for example by asking the following questions.

- How can we best prevent abuse?
- How can we identify when abuse has occurred and assess both the nature and extent of harm?
- When abuse is alleged or identified, how can we best manage the situation?
- Where people have been abused, how can we best support them on a short-term and long-term basis?

It is also important to remember that, in the context of healthcare, it is not only the patients and clients who may experience neglect and abuse: staff are also at risk. For example, Ferns and Meerabeau (2009) surveyed student nurses to determine their experience of verbal abuse. Forty-four per cent of the students who responded had experienced verbal abuse, mostly from patients, but some from visitors and other staff. Of those who disclosed that they had experienced abuse, 62.7 per cent said that they had reported such abuse, which means that 37.3 per cent had not reported the incident. The authors conclude that systems should be established to improve the reporting and documenting of verbal abuse that occurs during nurse education, and that support for students who experience abuse should be provided.

The challenges of researching safeguarding

It is important to undertake research about safeguarding issues. However, it can also be challenging. Key challenges relate to difficulties with definitions, the use of official statistics, and how best to determine 'success'. Each of these areas will be discussed.

The challenge of definition

The World Health Organization (WHO) (2002) includes abuse as part of its wider definition of violence, which views it as the intentional use of force or power that results in physical or psychological harm to self or others. Since WHO is a global organisation, it is to be expected that such a definition would influence many countries. However, if we take a critical look at this definition of violence, it can be seen that psychological abuse does not seem to be explicitly included and neither does financial abuse. Within England (DH, 2000a) and Wales (NAfW, 2000), psychological and financial abuse are included as recognised forms of abuse within policy guidance documents. However, while *In Safe Hands* (NAfW, 2000) and *No Secrets* (DH, 2000a) use the same definition of abuse, they categorise it in slightly different ways: the former refers to neglect, but the latter refers to neglect and acts of omission, and also includes discriminatory abuse. In Northern Ireland, a different definition of abuse is used (DHSSPS, 2006), but the same categories are used as in the English policy (DH, 2000a), with the addition of institutional abuse.

These examples show that how abuse is categorised and defined changes over time and between areas. In relation to research this can present us with two key difficulties. First, given that official definitions of what abuse is vary, it is likely that research participants will also have differing views as to what abuse is. Also, people will hold different views as to where, for example, bad practice ends and abuse begins. For example, some people would see a one-off incident as something that needs addressing, but if it recurred a number of times they would see it as abuse. As researchers, this means that we need to be very clear to define our terms carefully or, if we are trying to learn more about why abuse means different things to different people, we need to make sure we look carefully at the responses we get to identify both similarities and differences of views. The second difficulty arising from the use of different definitions is that it can make it difficult to compare studies from different countries, and also studies that occur at different times: even if the words used are the same, we may not be comparing like with like.

Using official statistics

The difficulties discussed above in relation to different definitions also apply to the use of official statistics and, therefore, caution is needed when using such information. Other challenges also exist in research when using data that have been recorded by services for the purpose of monitoring. Examples of such data include records of the numbers of people from different client groups who have been subject to alleged abuse. These data often include not only the client group and the type of alleged abuse, but also their relationship with the alleged perpetrators, and whether the allegations were proven or not proven.

The reliability of this information can, however, be challenged as a 'true' picture of the nature and extent of abuse. For example, not all abuse is reported. This can be for a number of reasons, including the fact that some people may not realise they have been abused, or they may not be able to communicate to others that they have been abused. They may be ashamed, or fear the consequences if they do report abuse, or they may not know who to report abuse to. Consider a young man with mental health problems who lives independently in the community and who is being sexually abused by a local youth. He reported this abuse but he was not believed and so now he feels it is not worth reporting it as no action was taken. Even though this is clearly an example of abuse, it will not feature in official statistics. When abuse is reported it may not always be acted upon in the same way, or may not be acted upon at all. For example, it was suggested earlier that people may use different thresholds to decide the point at which they feel they should treat something as abuse, and therefore their decisions as to whether or not to proceed using the official safeguarding procedure will vary (see the discussion regarding thresholds in Chapter 4, pages 70–2).

Abuse relating to one person may also take multiple forms, and this may not be easily understood from official data. For example, someone could be both financially and sexually abused. In this situation would it be possible to tell from the official statistics that these instances relate to the same person? Also, what about the person who is elderly and who also has learning disabilities – which client group should he or she be recorded in? If an elderly woman is abused by her husband, should this be recorded as domestic violence or as abuse? Finally, the way data are recorded can vary from one area to another, meaning that it is difficult to draw comparisons between areas. It can also be difficult to bring the data together to develop a broader data set.

Research about aspects such as numbers and types of referrals is important to see whether, and how, policies are being implemented. This means that issues such as those highlighted in the previous paragraph need to be carefully considered. Care also has to be taken when interpreting such information and Activity 10.5 encourages you to consider why this is the case.

Activity 10.5   *Critical thinking*

The Safeborough Health Trust implemented its safeguarding adults policy five years ago and now wants to evaluate its effectiveness. When it looks at the figures from the past five years, it finds that the numbers of allegations of abuse and neglect have increased each year. Some members of the management board are extremely worried by these results and think that the policy is failing or is not being implemented properly. However, others are pleased as they feel that the increase in allegations means that the policy is working well. Who is correct?

Suggestions are provided at the end of the chapter and in the discussion below.

How to determine success

Activity 10.5 asked you to consider two different interpretations of the same information. You may have found this challenging as both could be correct. If we look at the first view it is possible that, despite the existence of the policy, increasing incidents of abuse are occurring. This might suggest that staff are not aware of their responsibilities to protect patients from abuse and neglect, and more incidents are happening. However, it is also possible that, because of the policy, staff are more aware, feel more confident in recognising and addressing abuse, and therefore are more likely to report it. This would mean that an increase in reported incidents is an indication of success. The actual level of abuse may not have changed, but the level of reporting has. In reality, it would be important to investigate this information further to see whether other factors could have influenced the increase. For example, there could be issues such as changing patient characteristics, altered staffing levels, and other issues within the environment of care.

Another important issue to consider is who should determine whether or not safeguarding has been a success. Looking at official data may tell us one view of policy and practice development, but it does not tell us anything about how the process of safeguarding was experienced by those who have been abused or about how staff feel about the process. This is important to consider as, while the official policy might be viewed as a success in terms of due process being followed, and the policy-makers' outcome being achieved, the experience of those involved may have been very negative. In such circumstances, could the policy be seen to be a success? For example, in the review of *In Safe Hands* (Magill et al., 2010), people with learning disabilities said they were sometimes not believed and not kept informed if they reported abuse.

In determining success we also need to consider what the aim of the intervention or policy is: is it to prevent abuse, respond to abuse or to help people to recover from abuse? Total success in relation to safeguarding would mean that abuse and neglect do not occur, and that vulnerability is therefore reduced. However, it can be difficult to demonstrate that, by doing something such as adhering to a new policy, or by providing enhanced educational opportunities, some things (such as abuse and neglect) do not occur. Traditionally, research that wishes to explore the relationship between cause and effect uses an experimental approach. However, it would not be ethical to randomly assign patients or clients to groups in which the experimental group receives support from staff following the safeguarding policy, but the control group is supported by staff not following such a policy. It may therefore be more appropriate to undertake a before and after study in which a group acts as its own control. This would, however, mean that reliable data need to be collected before the intervention is started and, as noted above, such data in relation to safeguarding may be variable due to differing definitions and interpretations.

It would also be possible to research areas such as staff knowledge and attitudes that are relevant to safeguarding practice. For example, attitudes of staff working in A&E departments may vary in relation to people who self-harm and who then come to A&E. In such a situation there are clearly safeguarding issues as future episodes of self-harm could be life threatening. However, staff who view such patients as 'attention seeking' might dismiss them without recognising their distress. Alternatively, staff who are more empathetic might try to refer them to appropriate forms of support, even if they cannot provide support on a longer-term basis. A study examining staff attitudes may therefore be appropriate and might assist in developing educational interventions designed to promote more positive attitudes. Attitudes could then be reassessed to see if there has been any change.

Research that aims to determine nurses' knowledge of policy and legislation might also be relevant to safeguarding. For example, Chapter 6 discussed the relevance of the Mental Capacity Act 2005 to safeguarding, and research could be useful to discover the knowledge and under-standing that nurses have in relation to the law concerning capacity and consent, and how they use it in practice.

To determine the success of safeguarding measures we therefore need to consider carefully the following areas:

* the aims of the measures or interventions;
* who should determine success;
* how best to decide upon the appropriate research approach.

Each of these areas has ethical implications and therefore it is necessary to explore the ethics of research concerning safeguarding.

The ethics of safeguarding research

Research in relation to safeguarding is likely to focus on the experiences of groups often considered 'vulnerable subjects' in the context of research, and abuse and neglect are viewed as 'sensitive' topics. Each of these areas will be discussed.

Who is a 'vulnerable subject'?

People often considered to be 'vulnerable subjects' in research include those who have mental health problems, those who have learning disabilities, prisoners, people who are terminally ill, people with dementia and children. The fact that they are considered to be 'vulnerable' relates to a history that demonstrates the need for protection of research subjects (Juritzen et al., 2011). Well-known historical examples include the 'experiments' that were conducted on disabled people and other people in Nazi concentration camps during the Second World War, in which many of those experimented on suffered physical and psychological harm and, in some instances, death. Another example is the Tuskagee **syphilis** study, conducted in America between 1932 and 1972, which aimed to understand the course of untreated syphilis. During this longitudinal study, treatment for syphilis became available but was not given to study participants, who were black men from lower socio-economic backgrounds. The third study often quoted in this context is the Willowbrook Hospital study, conducted in the United States until the early 1970s. It took place in an overcrowded institution for children with learning disabilities. Conditions within the institution were very poor and viral **hepatitis** and other infections were prevalent. The researchers decided that they would allocate one ward specifically for the study of hepatitis and that they would deliberately infect children who were, with the consent of their parents, to be moved to this ward, where they could be studied with the aim of identifying a cure for hepatitis. They argued that the children would be at risk of contracting the infection wherever they were in the hospital and that by being on this ward they would be better cared for as they would be carefully studied.

The ethical issues within these examples relate to a lack of valid consent and the presence of coercion: for example, in the Nazi concentration camps those subjected to the experiments had no option of refusing. The researchers at Willowbrook presented an argument that the children would be at less risk taking part in the study than they would remaining on other wards, but nonetheless actively harmed the children by infecting them. Similarly, the participants in the Tuskagee study and the concentration camps suffered harm.

In response to these (and other) concerns, codes of ethical research practice were developed, and the need for review of proposed studies by ethics committees were established. Box 10.1 sets out some examples of such codes of, and guidelines for, research ethics. You may wish to compare and contrast their contents.

> **Box 10.1: Codes of research ethics**
>
> - World Medical Association (2008) *Declaration of Helsinki*
>   www.wma.net/en/30publications/10policies/b3/index.html
> This is an international code of biomedical ethics that is regularly reviewed and updated.
>
> - Royal College of Nursing (2009) *Research Ethics: RCN guidance for nurses*
>   www.rcn.org.uk/development/researchanddevelopment/rs/publications_and_
>   position_statements/research_ethics_guidance

This guidance is produced specifically for nurses undertaking research and those who use research.

- Economic and Social Research Council (2010) *Framework for Research Ethics* www.esrc.ac.uk/about-esrc/information/research-ethics.aspx

This guidance is produced by a leading funder of social science research.

- Social Research Association (2003) *Ethical Guidelines* http://the-sra.org.uk/wp-content/uploads/ethics03.pdf

This is another example of guidelines that relate to social science research.

The presence of such codes does not, however, ensure that people who might be vulnerable to harm, coercion or exploitation in the context of research are protected, and some authors express concern about applying the label 'vulnerable groups'. Levine et al. (2004) argue that it is applied to too many groups, which makes it meaningless, and also it stereotypes people within a group without considering individual characteristics that may (or may not) be relevant. The implications of this can be understood by considering the fact that some people may consider all people over the age of 80 to be 'vulnerable' research participants. However, while some people of this age may have difficulties in understanding information and giving consent, which would mean that special provisions might be needed if they were to take part in research, this would not be true of everyone of this age. Levine et al. (2004) also suggest that classifying people in this way may not protect them from harm.

This desire to 'protect' groups who are viewed as vulnerable from harm in research has led to some groups frequently being excluded from taking part in research or, if they are 'allowed' to be asked to take part, this can only happen if the permission of a professional 'gatekeeper' is obtained. In other words, they cannot be approached to take part unless a professional has given his or her approval for this to happen. This is not always welcomed by the potential participants. Ulivi et al. (2009) asked for mental health service users' views about access and consent for non-therapeutic research. Some viewed the requirement for the permission of a psychiatrist to be sought before they could be approached as 'offensive', and they saw no need for the psychiatrist to know if they were taking part in qualitative research.

Activity 10.6   *Reflection*

Imagine that you are a member of what is considered to be a 'vulnerable group' and you learn that other people have decided that you should not be asked to take part in a research study concerning discrimination and abuse within the health service.

- How do you think you would feel?
- Would you feel safeguarded?

As this activity is for your own reflection, there is no outline answer at the end of the chapter.

Juritzen et al. (2011) argue that 'vulnerable' groups of research participants can be vulnerable to another form of harm or offence due to their exclusion from research: by not participating in research their lives are not examined and made visible for public scrutiny, which can make them more vulnerable. Consider, for example, if researchers had not studied and exposed the conditions within some care settings. Poor standards of care and abuse would then have continued, because nobody outside the setting knew about them.

Discussing the situation of people with learning disabilities, McClimens and Allmark (2011) also argue that the emphasis on protecting them in the context of research has led to their exclusion. This, in turn, has led to many gaps in the evidence base relating to the support of people with learning disabilities because the research has not been undertaken. If this is applied to the specific situation of safeguarding from abuse and neglect, you can see how damaging this could be. Exclusion from research also means that 'vulnerable' groups can be subject to continued unacceptable practices and they may be denied the benefits of advances in care that have arisen from research (Juritzen et al., 2011).

So, we can see from the above that, while some people may be at greater risk of suffering harm in the context of research, harm can also occur as a result of being excluded from research. Liamputtong (2007) argues that this exclusion can increase vulnerability and Alexander (2010) suggests that it is unethical not to provide the opportunity for people to participate if they so wish, since to exclude them means that they are denied the potential benefits of research. These benefits could be wide ranging and include the direct impact of specific interventions, the more indirect benefits of improving care for others, and perhaps the personal benefits in terms of, for example, self-esteem.

The challenge is how best to safeguard potentially vulnerable research participants while also ensuring that they are able to participate if they so wish. This requires researchers to consider carefully how information is provided, how consent is obtained, how any harms can best be identified and minimised as much as possible, and how support is provided for participants should they experience any distress as a consequence of the research. Where the research focuses on abuse and neglect, however, there is another issue that has to be considered carefully: the subject itself is considered 'sensitive'.

What is a 'sensitive' topic?

Deciding what is considered to be 'sensitive' research can be difficult as what seems sensitive to one person may not be viewed in the same way by someone else, and only those who take part are really qualified to decide (Alexander, 2010). Topics not initially thought to be sensitive can, therefore, become sensitive in the course of fieldwork (Davison, 2004). In a study of adults who had been supported as children by child welfare services, Helgeland (2005) discussed ethical concerns with one participant. The participant pointed out that the concerns were those of researchers and that people like him, who had lived through difficult times, were grateful that someone cared enough to find out about their situation.

Some subjects are frequently considered to be sensitive, and these include death, violence and abuse (Dickson-Swift et al., 2008). However, these authors argue that not undertaking such research could be seen as an 'evasion of responsibility'. This means that, while there are ethical issues related to researching sensitive topics, there are also ethical implications that arise if decisions are taken not to do such research. Without such research our understanding of, for example, abuse will be limited, which means that our ability to prevent it, and respond to it effectively, will be seriously impaired.

Researchers undertaking sensitive research need to carefully consider the issues that may arise, the consequences of these issues, and the strategies that will be put in place to minimise their negative impact. For example, speaking with people about previous experiences of abuse may bring feelings to the surface that have been repressed for many years. Participants may become distressed, and it is important to anticipate this possibility, and to have support mechanisms such as counselling services in place should they be needed. Some may question whether such research should be undertaken as it could give rise to distress. An alternative view would be that the participants would be living with those feelings anyway, and it might be better to allow them to discuss them and to receive support. In addition, it is possible that their experiences may also bring wider benefits as they could enable a better understanding and the development of more appropriate support services.

Data collection and disclosure

A further issue that can arise is how to deal with disclosures of abuse during the process of data collection. This is a particular concern for nurses undertaking research as, even though they may be acting as researchers, they are still registered nurses and are therefore required to practise within the framework of their *Code* (NMC, 2008a). Before reading further, take a few minutes to read the following case study and to complete Activity 10.7.

Case study: Sue Wilson

Sue Wilson has just started working as a nurse researcher in a project that is exploring the experiences of mental health service users in relation to safeguarding from abuse within health service settings. During the course of an interview with a client at the day hospital the client tells her that, while he was an in-patient in the hospital, he was physically abused by a member of staff. He immediately says, however, that he does not want Sue to tell anyone and that she must promise that she will not tell anyone as everything they say in the interview is confidential. Sue has read the study protocol and knows that she should report this disclosure, but she feels under pressure to agree to keep the information to herself.

Activity 10.7   *Decision making and communication*

Imagine you are in Sue's position in the above situation.

- How would you respond to the disclosure and the pressure from the client to keep the information to yourself?
- How could the research be designed to make sure that participants are clearly informed that there are limits to confidentiality?
- How would you use your communication skills to assist you in this process?

Some suggestions are given at the end of the chapter.

It is also important to remember that sensitivities within research do not apply just to participants: researchers and others such as those who transcribe data can also be affected. It can be extremely difficult to listen to accounts of distressing and disturbing experiences and this can upset any researcher. It may also be that researchers have previous experiences of violence and abuse, and, while this may lead them to be interested in undertaking research in this area, it can also create emotional difficulties for them. A reflexive approach (see Chapter 7, page 143), the availability of supervision and support, and a willingness to use such support are therefore important for those undertaking research in relation to safeguarding.

An agenda for future research

Despite the challenges in undertaking research concerning safeguarding, it is essential that such research is both undertaken and widely disseminated, so that practice is regularly examined and improved. In developing future research there are a number of areas that need to be considered. First, as this book has shown, there are many different forms of abuse and neglect, and often individuals are subject to multiple forms of abuse. It is important that all of these are considered as to date some (for example, financial abuse) have tended to be under-researched. This is important to healthcare as (if the example of financial abuse is used) someone who has little or no money will have limited capacity to buy food, heat the house or clothe themselves adequately, and his or her health may be adversely affected.

It is also important that the diversity of people who experience abuse is reflected in future research. To date, much of the work that has been published has focused on the situation of older people and, to some extent, people with learning disabilities. Less work has been published that focuses on the situation, and experiences of, physically disabled people and those with mental health problems. It is also important to acknowledge that nurses themselves may be subjected to abuse in both work and private contexts: these areas require research attention so that they can be better understood and more effective supports can be provided.

It is important that all stages of the abuse and neglect trajectory are included. Preventing abuse and neglect needs to be a priority and we need to understand how this can be more effectively achieved. If abuse does occur, we need to understand what the barriers to effective policy implementation are and how these can be addressed. We need to evaluate the effectiveness of interventions provided to support people who have been abused, as in the current context of evidence-based care and value for money we need to demonstrate not only that something works, but also that the benefits achieved justify the costs.

Finally, it is essential that people who use health and social care services are involved in setting the agenda for research and are active partners in the research process. This is important if research is to be able to meet their self-defined needs and priorities.

These are, however, only some suggestions as to what might be included in a future research agenda. Since this is a relatively new area of practice, there is the potential for many develop-ments that need to be researched so that research informs practice, and policy and practice issues give rise to further research. Nurses must be fully engaged in the emerging safeguarding research agenda. If you are required to undertake a critical review of the literature for your dissertation, one way you might become involved in this is by focusing on an aspect of safeguarding for your topic.

Chapter summary

Safeguarding adults is a relatively new but important focus within research. Undertaking such research presents challenges in terms of the practical and ethical issues that can arise when researching what might be considered to be a 'sensitive' topic, with people who are viewed as being 'vulnerable'. However, not undertaking such research could make safeguarding practice less effective and therefore increase vulnerability. In recognising our professional responsibilities to safeguard those in our care we must recognise that, to do this, we need to engage in research both as critical consumers of other people's work, and as researchers in our own right.

Activities: Brief outline answers

Activity 10.1 Evidence-based practice and research, page 189

As you will have read in this chapter, nurses are required to base their practice on the best available evidence (NMC, 2008a). This means that, where it is available, appropriate research should be accessed, critically reviewed and used to inform the development of both individual practice and service provision. Broadly speaking, research is needed in relation to how best to prevent neglect, abuse and harm, how to respond to such events if they occur, and how to support people during and following these events. Also, given that abuse and neglect are not always recognised or reported at the time they occur, we also need research that helps us to better understand the long-term effects, since as health professionals we may meet patients and clients whose current difficulties are the result of events that occurred many years ago.

Activity 10.2 Evidence-based practice and research, page 191

Your answer to this activity will inevitably depend on the question you chose. However, to illustrate the issues you may have encountered, the example given in the activity will be used here. When identifying search terms, it is important to include not only those terms used in the question, but also terms that might be used to describe the same issue. For example, it would be important to use 'older adults' as a search term, but you would also need to use such terms as 'elderly' and 'elder'. You would need to include terms relating to nursing, safeguarding and physical abuse. However, it would be necessary to use other terms such as 'elder abuse', since this terminology is used widely, especially in the United States. The commonly used databases CiNAHL and Medline will be relevant. However, other databases such as ASSIA and PsychInfo would also be helpful. Using different databases is important as different journals are indexed with different databases. You may wish to set limits to your search in terms of dates, languages and countries.

Having undertaken your search you will probably find that you have a number of 'hits' that are not relevant to your chosen topic. For example, as soon as you include 'abuse' as a search term there is a tendency for databases to include papers that focus on substance misuse. Similarly, even where the term 'safeguarding' is used in conjunction with 'adults', databases still have a tendency to identify papers relating to children as safeguarding has a longer history with this client group. Another factor you will need to be alert to is the fact that individuals often experience multiple forms of abuse and therefore studies you identify may not just focus on physical abuse.

Activity 10.4 Critical thinking, page 193

Some areas you might have identified are:

* research that has been undertaken regarding safeguarding in other settings, for example:
  – social care settings
  – social work practice
  – medical practice
  – different countries
* nursing research that is not specifically related to safeguarding but has relevance to this area of care, for example:
  – dignity
  – vulnerability
  – post-traumatic stress disorder
  – risk and safety
  – use of restraint.

These are, however, only examples and you may have identified many more.

Activity 10.5 Critical thinking, page 196

The possible answers to this activity are discussed in the chapter but here it is important to remind you that, while this activity used a hypothetical example, it is important that you think critically about any data you are given about safeguarding. This includes both results within published studies and reports that include national or local service statistics. You need to think about possible different ways they could be interpreted and the validity of the claims (if any) that are being made based on the data given.

Activity 10.7 Decision making and communication, page 201

As a registered nurse Sue is professionally required to act on the disclosure she receives. Not only has she a duty to the person she is interviewing, but she also has a duty to the other patients who may still be being cared for by the staff member concerned. She will need to use her communication skills to handle the immediate situation by acknowledging what she has been told, expressing concern for the participant, but explaining that, as a registered nurse, she has a duty to report such incidents. She may also need to make sure that appropriate support is provided for the participant.

The possibility of this happening should have been made clear to all research participants before they consented to take part in the study. They should be informed in writing that, while their information will be kept confidential, there are limits to this and that, if they disclose that they or someone else is being harmed, there will be a duty to report the incident to the appropriate person. It can also be helpful to remind participants of this immediately before you start an interview or focus group. Once a disclosure has been made, the researcher needs to follow his or her local policy for reporting abuse and neglect. This means that researchers need to be aware of the contents of these policies and what needs to be done before commencing fieldwork.

Further reading

Aveyard, H and Sharp, P (2009) *A Beginner's Guide to Evidence Based Practice in Health and Social Care.* Maidenhead: McGraw Hill.

This book provides a very useful (and readable) introduction to evidence-based care. It is aimed at both pre-registration students and qualified nurses who are returning to study.

Dickson-Swift, V, James, EL and Liamputtong, P (2008) *Undertaking Sensitive Research in the Health and Social Sciences: Managing boundaries, emotions and risks.* Cambridge: Cambridge University Press.

This book explores the issues that need to be considered by researchers undertaking sensitive research, both in relation to potential participants and in terms of their own well-being.

Liamputtong, P (2007) *Researching the Vulnerable.* London: Sage.

Ethical, moral and methodological issues relating to research with people who may be vulnerable are explored in this book.

Parkin, P (2009) *Managing Change in Healthcare: Using action research.* London: Sage.

This book introduces you to different approaches to change management but considers them within the context of the health service.

Useful websites

www.mind.org.uk/campaigns_and_issues/current_campaigns/another_assault/adult_safeguarding

This website contains research undertaken by MIND relating to safeguarding issues and people with mental health problems.

www.scie.org.uk

The Social Care Institute for Excellence provides a useful resource in terms of published research and research in progress, some of which relates to safeguarding.

www.who.int/violence_injury_prevention/violence/elder_abuse/en/index.html

This provides a link to the WHO pages that focus on the prevention of violence and abuse against older people. The materials you can access here will give you an international perspective on this subject.

Glossary

advocate   a person who undertakes to speak or campaign on behalf of another person, especially if the latter lacks the *capacity* or opportunity to speak for themselves.

attention deficit hyperactivity disorder (ADHD)   a behavioural disorder, especially of children, characterised by poor concentration and impulsive behaviour.

autistic spectrum   a wide range of developmental disorders, characterised by an inability to form normal social relationships, impairment of communication skills and an inability to understand abstract concepts.

autonomy   having control over your own life and making your own decisions without undue pressure from others; similar to *self-determination*.

beneficence   action undertaken that benefits others; doing good.

best interests   This is a phrase that is used generally to refer to situations where other people act in what they believe to be the best interests of another. See also *paternalism*. However, it also has a specific meaning within the Mental Capacity Act where it refers to the actions that should be taken when an individual lacks capacity to make a specific decision.

bipolar disorder   a mood disorder characterised by alternating manic and depressive periods; previously known as manic depression.

buggery   anal intercourse; it is also known as sodomy.

capacity   in the context of this book, this refers to a person's legal competence and ability to understand options and make decisions regarding his or her own welfare.

case law see common law

chemotherapy   a range of treatments usually given for cancer.

civil rights   the non-political rights of citizens of a country to live in freedom and enjoy social equality.

coercion   making someone do something against his or her will by using force or threats.

cognitive   relating to thinking and reasoning.

cognitive behavioural therapy (CBT)   a form of psychotherapy that aims to treat illnesses such as depression by helping the sufferer to replace negative thoughts and behaviours with desirable and positive ones.

common law (case law)   in England, the body of law relating to previous cases, customs and precedents, instead of *statutes*.

compassion   sympathy or *empathy* for the circumstances and suffering of others with a desire to improve matters.

confidentiality   in the context of nursing, keeping information private that has been entrusted to you by a patient.

consensus   general agreement; in nursing, this may have been reached by various research studies all coming to the same conclusion or by professional agreement.

consent   authorisation given to a nurse by a patient to carry out certain medical procedures. Adults are assumed to have the *capacity* to give or withhold consent unless assessed as lacking capacity. A *best interests* decision would then need to be taken.

dementia   used to describe any of a range of progressive mental disorders, usually affecting older people, such as Alzheimer's disease, characterised by deteriorating *cognitive* function, and physical health problems.

detention   in the context of this book, compulsorily admitting a person for assessment or treatment, for example under the Mental Health Act 1983.

diagnostic overshadowing   a form of *discrimination*, especially against people with learning disabilities and those with mental health problems, where all illnesses and symptoms are viewed as part of the learning disability or mental health problem and therefore they are not investigated as thoroughly as they would be in other people.

discrimination   making unjust or untrue assumptions about categories of people and treating them differently, especially unfavourably; see also *prejudice*.

Down's syndrome   a congenital chromosomal abnormality causing intellectual impairment and specific physical characteristics.

duty of care   a duty or responsibility owed to another person to look after him or her and not to do harm or increase his or her suffering.

dyslexia   difficulty in interpreting words and other symbols and learning to read and write; the numerical equivalent is called dyscalculia.

electroconvulsive therapy (ECT)   treating depression by applying electric shocks to certain areas of the brain.

empathy   understanding, being sensitive to and, in some cases, sharing the feelings and thoughts of others, even if they haven't been explicitly described to you.

epilepsy   a neurological disorder characterised by abnormal electrical discharges in the brain, resulting in seizures, loss of consciousness or sensory disturbance.

harassment   tormenting someone persistently, especially by unwelcome physical intimidation or verbal abuse.

hepatitis   a disease characterised by inflammation of the liver, some forms of which can be fatal.

hierarchy   a ranking system that puts what is perceived to be the most important at the top and what is perceived to be the least important at the bottom.

hospital passport   a document often used by people with learning disabilities that provides personal details, past medical history and likes and dislikes, and that describes how an individual should be treated. Its purpose is to assist communication with the individual and to promote care that meets his or her needs.

human rights   rights that are believed to belong fundamentally to all people, by virtue of being human.

incest   sexual relations between people who are too closely related, such as a brother and sister, or a father and daughter.

Independent Mental Capacity Advocate (IMCA)   an *advocate* who helps people who lack *capacity* and who do not have family members to support them when important decisions have to be taken regarding their medical treatment and other major life changes.

ischaemia   an inadequate blood supply to a body part, such as the heart or brain, due to an obstruction in the inflow of arterial blood.

justice   an ethical principle that is concerned with treating others fairly and ensuring equality and entitlement. Views regarding justice may differ according to culture, religion and moral values.

motivation   this is a factor that causes a person to act in a particular way. For example, in the context of abuse, a person could be motivated to act abusively towards others because he or she was abused as a child.

multiple sclerosis   a chronic, progressive disease marked by damage to the sheaths of nerve cells in the brain or spinal cord, resulting in paralysis, muscle tremors, speech impairment and blurred vision.

nebuliser a device for producing a fine spray of medication, so that it can be inhaled; it is especially used by those with asthma and other respiratory conditions.

non-maleficence the ethical principle of not harming others.

non-verbal communication also known as body language, this includes facial expressions, hand gestures, eye movements and body positions, such as crossing one's arms or leaning forward to listen to someone.

palliative care care that eases symptoms and reduces pain but that doesn't cure the disease itself; it is usually given to those in the final stages of terminal illnesses such as cancer.

paternalism making decisions for, or restricting the freedom and responsibilities of, other people in the belief that you are acting in their (supposed) *best interests*.

persecution similar to *harassment*, this is subjecting someone to prolonged hostility and ill-treatment, especially if they belong to a different social or religious group.

pindown a method of punishment where children were locked in rooms called 'pindown rooms', with little furniture and in solitary confinement, sometimes for weeks or months, with no conversation and repetitive occupations.

POVA An abbreviation often used as a shorthand to refer to the process known as 'Protection of vulnerable adults' that sets out what should occur when allegations of abuse are reported.

prejudice unjust behaviour towards, or an adverse opinion of, a person based on perceived, but not necessarily true, characteristics; for example, treating all old people as if they are mentally impaired.

psychosurgery brain surgery used to treat mental disorders.

qualitative research research involving such methods as interviews, focus groups and observations of people in their natural settings, in order to find out why and how people behave the way they do; it is contrasted with quantitative research, which gathers statistical data.

reasonable adjustments these are adjustments that service providers and employers are required by law to make to enable disabled people to access goods, services and employment on an equal basis as non-disabled people. These may be adjustments to, for example, the environment, the provision of information or to working arrangements.

resilience the ability to endure or recover quickly from difficult situations or unpleasant experiences.

self-determination the ability and freedom to control, or make decisions about, one's own life, without undue interference from other people; similar to *autonomy*.

statutes the laws established by the European Union, the UK Parliament and, increasingly, the devolved administrations of the countries of the UK, with which citizens must comply; see also *common law (case law)*.

stigma a mark of shame or disgrace; to stigmatise someone is to treat him or her as if they were worthy of disgrace.

syphilis a sexually transmitted, chronic and contagious disease that, if untreated, can affect the bones, muscles and brain.

therapeutic relationship the relationship between a nurse and his or her patient, which is important to the therapeutic process and to the well-being of both parties.

venflon a venous catheter (a small, flexible tube) placed into a peripheral vein in order to administer medication or fluids.

References

ACAS (2010) *Bullying and Harassment at Work: A guide for managers and employers.* Available online at www.acas.org.uk/CHttpHandler.ashx?id=304&p=0 (accessed 5 March 2012).

Action on Elder Abuse (2012) *Neglect.* Available online at www.elderabuse.org.uk/abuse_neglect.html (accessed 31 March 2012).

Ahern, K and McDonald, S (2002) The beliefs of nurses who were involved in a whistleblowing event. *Journal of Advanced Nursing,* 38(3): 303–9.

Alaszewski, A and Alaszewski, H (2011) Positive risk taking, in Atherton, H and Crickmore, D (eds) *Learning Disabilities: Toward inclusion,* 6th edition. Edinburgh: Churchill Livingstone, pp179–95.

Alexander, SJ (2010) 'As long as it helps somebody': why vulnerable people participate in research. *International Journal of Palliative Nursing,* 16(4): 173–8.

Association of Directors of Social Services (ADSS) (2005) *Safeguarding Adults.* London: ADSS. Available online at www.elderabuse.org.uk/Documents/ADASS%20guide%20-%20SAFEGUARDING%20 ADULTS.pdf (accessed 20 October 2012).

Atkinson, M, Jones, M and Lamont, E (2007) *Multi-agency Working and its Implications for Practice: A review of the literature.* Available online at www.nfer.ac.uk/nfer/publications/MAD01/MAD01.pdf (accessed 2 June 2012).

Aveyard, H and Sharp, P (2009) *A Beginner's Guide to Evidence Based Practice in Health and Social Care.* Maidenhead: Open University Press.

Aylett, J (2008) Learning the lessons in training from abuse inquiries: findings and recommendations. *Journal of Adult Protection,* 10(4): 7–11.

Backer, C, Chapman, M and Mitchell, D (2009) Access to secondary healthcare for people with intellectual disabilities: a review of the literature. *Journal of Applied Research in Intellectual Disabilities,* 22(6): 514–25.

Barker, P (2012) Ethics: in search of the good life, in Barker, P (ed.) *Mental Health Ethics: The human context.* London: Routledge, pp5–30.

Barr, H (2001) A review. Inter-professional education: today and tomorrow. Learning and Teaching Support Network Centre for Health Sciences and Practice. Available online at: www.heacademy.ac.uk/assets/ documents/subjects/health/occp/revised.pdf

BBC News (2011) News, 17 August. Available online at www.bbc.co.uk/news/uk-england-birmingham-14563038 (accessed 3 June 2012).

Beadle-Brown, J, Mansell, J, Cambridge, P, Milne, A and Whelton, B (2010) Adult protection of people with intellectual disabilities: incidence, nature and responses. *Journal of Applied Research in Intellectual Disabilities,* 23(6): 573–84.

Beauchamp, TL and Childress, JF (2009) *Principles of Biomedical Ethics,* 6th edition. New York: Oxford University Press.

Benbow, SM (2008) Failure in the system: our inability to learn from inquiries. *Journal of Adult Protection,* 10(3): 5–13.

Berry, LE (2011) Creating community: strengthening education and practice partnerships through communities of practice. *International Journal of Nursing Education Scholarship,* 8(1): 1–18.

Bond, M and Holland, S (2010) *Skills of Clinical Supervision for Nurses: A practical guide for supervisees, clinical supervisors and managers,* 2nd edition. Maidenhead: Open University Press.

Braye, S, Orr, D and Preston-Shoot, M (2011) Conceptualising and responding to self-neglect: the challenges for adult safeguarding. *Journal of Adult Protection,* 13(4): 182–93.

British Medical Association (BMA) (2011) *Safeguarding Vulnerable Adults: A toolkit for general practitioners.* London: BMA.

Brown, H (1999) Abuse of people with learning disabilities, in Stanley, N, Manthorpe, J and Penhale, B (eds) *Institutional Abuse: Perspectives across the life course.* London: Routledge, pp89–109.

Buka, P (2008) *Patients' Rights, Law and Ethics for Nurses,* London: Hodder Arnold.

Burke, L, Lopez, J and Treadwell, E (2009) Social policy, in Sines, D, Saunders, M and Forbes-Burford, J (eds) *Community Health Care Nursing*, Oxford: Blackwell Science, pp17–32.

Buzgova, R and Ivanova, K (2011) Violation of ethical principles in institutional care for older people, *Nursing Ethics*, 18(1): 64–78.

Care Quality Commission (CQC) (2010) *Essential Standards of Quality and Safety*. London: CQC.

Care Quality Commission (CQC) (2012) *Learning Disability Services Inspection Programme: National overview*. Newcastle Upon Tyne: CQC.

Chandler, L and Fry, A (2009) Can communities of practice make a meaningful contribution to sustainable service improvement in health and social care? *Journal of Integrated Care*, 17(2): 41–8.

Clarke, HF and Driever, MJ (1983) Vulnerability: the development of a construct for nursing, in Chinn, PL (ed.) *Advances in Nursing Theory Development*, Gaithersberg, MD: Aspen.

College and Association of Registered Nurses of Alberta (CARNA) (2005) *Position Statement on Vulnerability*, Edmonton: CARNA.

Collins, M (2010) Thresholds in adult protection. *Journal of Adult Protection*, 12(1): 4–12.

Commission for Social Care Inspection (CSCI) (2008) *Safeguarding Adults: A study of the effectiveness of arrangements to safeguard adults from abuse*. Newcastle: CSCI.

Committee of Inquiry (1969) *Report of the Committee of Inquiry into Allegations of Ill-treatment of Patients and other Irregularities at the Ely Hospital, Cardiff*, Cmd 3975. London: HMSO.

Crown Prosecution Service (CPS) (2012a) Fact sheet on hate crime. Available online at www.cps.gov.uk/news/fact_sheets/hate_crime/ (accessed 26 March 2012).

Crown Prosecution Service (CPS) (2012b) *Hate Crime and Crimes against Older People Report 2010–2011*. Available online at www.cps.gov.uk/publications/docs/cps_hate_crime_report_2011.pdf (accessed 27 March 2012).

Currie, L and Loftus-Hills, A (2002) The nursing view of clinical governance. *Nursing Standard*, 16(27): 40–4.

Daily Mail (2009) Starved to death in an NHS hospital: damning inquiry highlights case of patient left without food for 26 days. Available online at www.dailymail.co.uk/news/article-1110054/Starved-death-NHS-hospital-Damning-inquiry-highlights-case-patient-left-food-26-days.html#ixzz1q L9ZKKBH (accessed 5 May 2012).

D'Amour, D, Ferrada-Videla, M, San Martin Rodriguez, L and Beaulieu, MD (2005) The conceptual basis for interprofessional collaboration: core concepts and theoretical frameworks. *Journal of Interprofessional Care*, 19: 116–31.

Davies, R and Jenkins R (2004) Preventing abuse and protecting clients: a key role for the learning disability nurse. *Journal of Adult Protection*, 6(2): 31–41.

Davies, R, Llewellyn, P, Sardi, I, Netana, C, Stackhouse, B, Jenkins, R, Collins, M and Kay, A (2009) *The Experience of Vulnerable Adults: Adult protection practice*. Pontypridd: University of Glamorgan.

Davies, R, Collins, M, Netana, C, Folkes, L, Jenkins, R, Tombs, M, Kaye, A, Stackhouse, B and Evans, C (2011) *Exploring the Motivations of Perpetrators who Abuse Vulnerable Adults*. Newport: University of Wales.

Davison, J (2004) Dilemmas in research: issues of vulnerability and disempowerment for the social worker/researcher. *Journal of Social Work Practice*, 18(3): 379–93.

Deacon, J (1982) *Tongue Tied: Fifty years of friendship in a subnormality hospital*. London: Royal Society for Mentally Handicapped Children and Adults.

Delor, F and Hubert, M (2000) Revisiting the concept of 'vulnerability'. *Social Science and Medicine*, 50: 1557–70.

Department of Constitutional Affairs (2007) *Mental Capacity Act 2005 Code of Practice (2007 Final Edition)*. London: The Stationery Office.

Department of Health (DH) (1997) *The New NHS: Modern, dependable*. London: HMSO.

Department of Health (DH) (1998) *A First Class Service: Quality in the new NHS health services*. London: HMSO.

Department of Health (DH) (1999a) *National Service Framework for Mental Health: Modern standards and service models*. London: Department of Health.

Department of Health (DH) (1999b) *Clinical Governance: Quality in the new NHS*. London: HMSO.

Department of Health (DH) (2000a) *No Secrets: Guidance on developing and implementing multi-agency policies and procedures to protect vulnerable adults from abuse*. London: The Stationery Office.

Department of Health (DH) (2000b) *The NHS Plan.* London: Department of Health.

Department of Health (DH) (2001) *Modern Standards and Service Models: National Service Framework for Older People.* London: Department of Health.

Department of Health (DH) (2003) *Confidentiality: NHS code of practice,* London: Department of Health.

Department of Health (DH) (2007) *Best Practice in Managing Risk: Principles and guidance for best practice in the assessment and management of risk to self and others in mental health services.* London: Department of Health.

Department of Health (DH) (2008) *Human Rights in Healthcare: A framework for local action,* 2nd edition. London: Department of Health.

Department of Health (DH) (2009a) *Living Well with Dementia: A national dementia strategy.* London: Department of Health.

Department of Health (DH) (2009b) *Safeguarding Adults: Report on the consultation on the review of 'No Secrets'.* London: Department of Health.

Department of Health (DH) (2009c) *Valuing People Now: A new three-year strategy for people with learning disabilities.* London: Department of Health.

Department of Health (DH) (2010a) *Clinical Governance and Adult Safeguarding: An integrated process.* London: Department of Health.

Department of Health (DH) (2010b) *Essence of Care 2010.* London: Department of Health.

Department of Health (DH) (2010c) *Supplementary Guidance: Public interest disclosure.* London: Department of Health.

Department of Health (DH) (2011a) *Safeguarding Adults: The role of health service practitioners.* London: Department of Health.

Department of Health (DH) (2011b) What is clinical governance? Available online at www.dh.gov.uk/health/2011/09/clinical-governance/ (accessed 10 June 2012).

Department of Health, Social Services and Public Safety (DHSSPS) (2006) *Safeguarding Vulnerable Adults. Regional adult protection policy and procedural guidance.* Ballymena: NHSSB.

Department of Health, Social Services and Public Safety (2010) *Adult Safeguarding in Northern Ireland: Regional and local partnership arrangements.* Belfast: Northern Ireland Office.

De Santis, J (2008) Exploring the concepts of vulnerability and resilience in the context of HIV infection. *Research and Theory for Nursing Practice,* 22(4): 273–87.

Dickson-Swift, V, James, EL and Liamputtong, P (2008) *Undertaking Sensitive Research in the Health and Social Sciences.* Cambridge: Cambridge University Press.

Disability Rights Commission (DRC) (2006) *Part 1. Equal Treatment: Closing the Gap: A formal investigation into the physical health inequalities experienced by people with learning disabilities and/or mental health problems.* London: Disability Rights Commission.

Domestic Violence (2012) What is domestic violence? Available online at www.domesticviolence.co.uk/ (accessed 1 April 2012).

Dougherty, L and Lister, S (eds) (2011) *The Royal Marsden Hospital Manual for Clinical Procedures: Student edition,* 8th edition. Chichester: Wiley-Blackwell.

Draper, T, Roots, S and Carter, H (2009) Safeguarding adults: perspectives from primary care trusts in Kent and Medway. *Journal of Adult Protection,* 11(3): 6–11.

Edwards, SD (2009) *Nursing Ethics: A principle based approach,* 2nd edition. Basingstoke: Palgrave Macmillan.

Erdil, F and Korkmaz, F (2009) Ethical problems observed by student nurses. *Nursing Ethics,* 16(5): 589–98.

Ferns, T and Meerabeau, E (2009) Reporting behaviours of nursing students who have experienced verbal abuse. *Journal of Advanced Nursing,* 65(12): 2678–88.

Flaskerud, JH and Winslow, BW (2010) Vulnerable populations and ultimate responsibility. *Issues in Mental Health Nursing,* 31: 298–9.

Firtko, A and Jackson, D (2005) Do the ends justify the means? Nursing and the dilemma of whistleblowing. *Australian Journal of Advanced Nursing,* 23(1): 51–6.

Francis, R (2010) *Independent Inquiry into Care Provided by Mid Staffordshire NHS Foundation Trust January 2005–March 2009, Volumes 1 and 2.* London: The Stationery Office.

Fry, ST and Johnstone, M (2008) *Ethics in Nursing Practice: A guide to ethical decision making.* Oxford: Blackwell Publishing.

Fyson, R and Kitson, R (2010) Human rights and social wrongs: issues in safeguarding adults with learning disabilities. *Practice: Social Work in Action*, 22(5): 309–20.

Goffman, E (1961) *Asylums: Essays on the social situation of mental patients and other inmates*. New York: Doubleday.

Grealish, L, Bail, K and Ranse, K (2010) 'Investing in the future': residential aged care staff experiences of working with nursing students in a 'community of practice'. *Journal of Clinical Nursing*, 19: 2291–9.

Griffith, R and Tengnah, C (2010) *Law and Professional Issues in Nursing*, 2nd edition. Exeter: Learning Matters.

The Guardian Tuesday (2011) Fiona Pilkington case, 24 May. Available online at]www.guardian.co.uk/uk/2011/may/24/fiona-pilkington-police-misconduct-proceedings (accessed 20 June 2012).

Health and Safety Executive (HSE) (2007) *Managing the Causes of Work-related Stress: A step-by-step approach using the management standards*, 2nd edition. London: The Stationery Office.

Health and Safety Executive (HSE) (2011a) *Five Steps to Risk Assessment*. Available online at www.hse.gov.uk/pubns/indg163.pdf (accessed 24 June 2012).

Health and Safety Executive (HSE) (2011b) *Stress and Psychological Disorders*. Available online at www.hse.gov.uk/statistics/causdis/stress/stress.pdf (accessed 25 June 2012).

Healthcare Commission (HCC) (2006) *Joint Investigation into the Provision of Services for People with Learning Disabilities at Cornwall Partnership NHS Trust*. London: Commission for Healthcare Audit and Inspection.

Health Inspectorate Wales (HIW) (2010) *Safeguarding and Protecting Vulnerable Adults in Wales: A review of the arrangements in place across the Welsh National Health Service*. Caerphilly: Health Inspectorate Wales.

Helgeland, IM (2005) 'Catch 22' of research ethics: ethical dilemmas in follow-up studies of marginal groups. *Qualitative Inquiry*, 11(4): 549–69.

Hill, M (2009) *The Public Policy Process*, 5th edition. Harlow: Pearson Longman.

Hoffmaster, B (2006) What does vulnerability mean? *Hastings Center Report*, 36(2): 38–45.

House of Commons Select Committee (2007) *Elder Abuse: Second report of the session 2003–04, vol. 1*. London: The Stationery Office.

Jack, R (1998) Institutions in community care, in Jack, R (ed.) *Residential Versus Community Care: The role of institutions in welfare provision*. Basingstoke: Macmillan, pp10–40.

Jenkins, R (1997) Issues of empowerment for nurses and clients. *Nursing Standard*, 11(46): 44–6.

Jenkins, R (2009) Older people with learning disabilities: a quality initiative in caring, in Froggatt, K, Davies, S and Meyer, J (eds) *Understanding Care Homes: A research and development perspective*. London: Jessica Kingsley, pp91–110.

Jenkins, R and Davies, R (2004) The abuse of adults with learning disabilities and the role of the learning disability nurse. *Learning Disability Practice*, 7(2): 30–8.

Jenkins, R and Davies, R (2006) Neglect of people with intellectual disabilities: a failure to act? *Journal of Intellectual Disabilities*, 10(1): 35–45.

Jenkins, R, Davies, R and Northway, R (2008) Zero tolerance of abuse of people with learning disabilities: implications for nursing. *Journal of Clinical Nursing*, 17(22): 3041–9.

Johnson, DE (1990) The behavioural system model for nursing, in Parker, ME (ed.) *Nursing Theories in Practice*. New York: National League for Nursing.

Juritzen, TI, Grimen, H and Heggen, K (2011) Protecting vulnerable research participants: a Foucault-inspired analysis of ethics committees. *Nursing Ethics*, 18(3): 640–50.

Kesson, EM, Allardice, GM, George, D, Burns, HJG and Morrison, DS (2012) Effects of multidisciplinary team working on breast cancer survival: retrospective, comparative, interventional cohort study of 13,722 women. *British Medical Journal*. Available online at www.bmj.com/highwire/filestream/581371/field_highwire_article_pdf/0.pdf (accessed 24 May 2012).

Kvarnström, S (2008) Difficulties in collaboration: a critical incident study of interprofessional healthcare teamwork. *Journal of Interprofessional Care*, 22(2): 191–203.

Lawson, HA (2004) The logic of collaboration in education and the human services. *Journal of Interprofessional Care*, 18(3): 225–37.

Lees, A and Meyer, E (2011) Theoretically speaking: use of a communities of practice framework to describe and evaluate interprofessional education. *Journal of Interprofessional Care*, 25: 84–90.

Levine, C, Faden, R, Grady, C, Hammerschmidt, D, Eckenwiler, L and Sugarman, J (2004) The limitations of 'vulnerability' as a protection for human research participants. *The American Journal of Bioethics*, 4(3): 44–9.

Liamputtong, P (2007) *Researching the Vulnerable*. London: Sage.

Lipp, A (2004) Reflexivity: a method of research and professional development. *Journal of Advanced Perioperative Care*, 2(2): 55–8.

Lo, KLL, Lai, CKY and Tsui, CM (2009) Student nurses' perception and understanding of elder abuse. *International Journal of Older People Nursing*, 5: 283–9.

Magill, J, Yeates, B and Longley, M (2010) *Review of In Safe Hands: A review of the Welsh Assembly government's guidance on the protection of vulnerable adults in Wales*. Pontypridd: University of Glamorgan.

Malone, RE (2000) Dimensions of vulnerability in emergency nurses' narratives. *Advances in Nursing Science*, 23(1): 1–11.

Mantell, A (2008) Human rights and wrongs: the Human Rights Act 1998, in Mantell, A and Scragg, T (eds) *Safeguarding Adults in Social Work*. Exeter: Learning Matters, pp31–43.

Manthorpe, J (1999) Users' perceptions: searching for the views of users with learning disabilities, in Stanley, N, Manthorpe, J and Penhale, B (eds) *Institutional Abuse: Perspectives across the life course*. London: Routledge, pp110–29.

Manthorpe, J and Stanley, N (1999) Shifting the focus: from 'bad apples' to users' rights, in Stanley, N, Manthorpe, J and Penhale, B (eds) *Institutional Abuse: Perspectives across the life course*. London: Routledge, pp223–40.

Marsland, D, Oakes, P and White, C (2007) Abuse in care? The identification of early indicators of the abuse of people with learning disabilities in residential settings. *Journal of Adult Protection*, 9(4): 6–20.

Martin, J (2007) *Safeguarding Adults*. Lyme Regis: Russell House.

Mathias, P and Thompson, T (2001) Interprofessional and multi-agency working, in Thompson, J and Pickering, S (eds) *Meeting the Health Needs of People Who Have a Learning Disability*, Edinburgh: Bailliere Tindall, pp320–35.

McCallin, A (2001) Interdisciplinary practice – a matter of teamwork: an integrated literature review. *Journal of Clinical Nursing*, 10(4): 419–28.

McClimens, A and Allmark, P (2011) A problem with inclusion in learning disability research. *Nursing Ethics*, 18(5): 633–9.

McConkey, R (2007) Leisure and work, in Gates, B (ed.) *Learning Disabilities Toward Inclusion*, 5th edition. Edinburgh: Churchill Livingstone, pp169–88.

McDonald, A (2010) The impact of the 2005 Mental Capacity Act on social workers' decision making and approaches to the assessment of risk. *British Journal of Social Work*, 40: 1229–46.

McGarry, J, Simpson, C and Hinchliff-Smith, K (2011) The impact of domestic abuse for older women: a review of the literature. *Health and Social Care in the Community*, 19(1): 3–14.

McKay, E, Ryan, S and Sumsion, T (2003) Three journeys towards reflexivity, in Finlay, L and Gough, B (eds) *Reflexivity: A practical guide for researchers in health and social sciences*. Oxford: Blackwell, pp52–65.

McVicar, A (2003) Workplace stress in nursing: a literature review. *Journal of Advanced Nursing*, 44(6): 633–42.

Mencap (2004) *Treat Me Right: Better healthcare for people with a learning disability*. London: Mencap.

Mencap (2007) *Death by Indifference: Following up the Treat Me Right report*. London: Mencap.

Mencap (2012) *Death by Indifference: 74 deaths and counting. A progress report 5 years on*. London: Mencap.

Merrell, J, Philpin, S, Warring, J, Hobby, D and Gregory, V (2012) Addressing the nutritional needs of older people in residential care homes. *Health & Social Care in the Community*, 20(2): 208–15.

Michaels, J (2008) *Report of the Independent Inquiry into Access to Healthcare for People with Learning Disabilities*. Available online at www.dh.gov.uk/prod_consum_dh/groups/dh_digitalassets/@dh/@en/documents/digitalasset/dh_106126.pdf (accessed 20 February 2012).

Mind (2007) *Chance Could Be a Fine Thing: Reassessing risk in mental health*. London: Mind.

Molyneux, J (2001) Interprofessional teamworking: what makes teams work well? *Journal of Inter-professional Care*, 15(1): 29–35.

Morgan, A (2010) Review of safeguarding practice points towards a new culture of transparency. *Nursing Older People*, 22(1): 6–7.

Mornington, JM and Mornington, M (2008) Domestic violence and honour based crime: joined up governance and an Islamic approach, in Pritchard, J (ed.) *Good Practice in Safeguarding Adults.* London: Jessica Kingsley, pp65–82.

National Assembly for Wales (NAfW) (2000) *In Safe Hands: Protection of vulnerable adults in Wales.* Cardiff, NafW.

National Patient Safety Agency (NPSA) (2008) *A Risk Matrix for Risk Managers.* London: NPSA. Available online at www.npsa.nhs.uk/nrls/improvingpatientsafety/patient-safety-tools-and-guidance/risk-assessment-guides/risk-matrix-for-risk-managers/ (accessed 16 October 2012).

Nazarko, L (2001) See, hear – then speak out. *Nursing Standard*, 15(20): 22.

Neuman, B (1995) *The Neuman Systems Model.* Norwalk, CT: Appleton & Lange.

NHS Executive (1994) *Risk Management in the NHS.* London: Department of Health.

Northway, R and Jenkins, R (2007) Specialist learning disability services, in Gates, B (ed.) *Learning Disabilities: Toward inclusion*, 5th edition. Edinburgh: Churchill Livingstone, pp105–23.

Northway, R, Davies, R, Mansell, I and Jenkins, R (2007) 'Policies don't protect people, it's how they are implemented': policy and practice in protecting people with learning disabilities from abuse. *Social Policy and Administration*, 41(1): 86–104.

Nursing and Midwifery Council (NMC) (2002) *Practitioner–Client Relationships and the Prevention of Abuse.* London: NMC.

Nursing and Midwifery Council (NMC) (2008a) *The Code: Standards of conduct, performance and ethics for nurses and midwives.* London: NMC.

Nursing and Midwifery Council (NMC) (2008b) *Clinical Supervision for Registered Nurses.* Available online at www.nmc-uk.org/Nurses-and-midwives/Advice-by-topic/A/Advice/Clinical-supervision-for-registered-nurses/ (accessed 9 May 2012).

Nursing and Midwifery Council (NMC) (2009) Confidentiality advice. Available online at www.nmc-uk.org/Nurses-and-midwives/Advice-by-topic/A/Advice/Confidentiality/ (accessed 25 April 2012).

Nursing and Midwifery Council (NMC) (2010a) Fact sheet. Available online at www.nmc-uk.org/Documents/Safeguarding/Toolkit/FACT%20SHEET_Safeguarding%20adults.pdf (accessed 25th February 2012).

Nursing and Midwifery Council (NMC) (2010b) *Raising and Escalating Concerns: Guidance for nurses and midwives.* London: NMC.

Nursing and Midwifery Council (NMC) (2010c) *Standards for Pre-registration Nursing Education.* London: NMC.

Nursing and Midwifery Council (NMC) (2011) *Nursing and Midwifery Council: Annual fitness to practise report 2010–2011.* London: The Stationery Office.

The Observer (2010) More than 40% of domestic violence victims are male, report reveals. Available online at www.guardian.co.uk/society/2010/sep/05/men-victims-domestic-violence (accessed 25 May 2012).

O'Callaghan, AC, Murphy, G and Clare, ICH (2003) The impact of abuse on men and women with severe learning disabilities and their families. *British Journal of Learning Disabilities*, 31: 175–80.

O'Keeffe, M, Hills, A, Doyle, M, McCreadie, C, Scholes, S, Constantine, R, Tinker, A, Manthorpe, J, Biggs, S and Erens, B (2007) *UK Study of Abuse and Neglect of Older People Prevalence Survey Report.* London: National Centre for Social Research.

Older People's Commissioner for Wales (2010) *'Dignified Care': The experiences of older people in hospital in Wales.* Cardiff: The Older People's Commissioner for Wales.

Older People's Commissioner for Wales (2012) *Dignified Care Responses.* Available online at www.olderpeoplewales.com/en/Reviews/dignity-and-respect/Hospital-review.aspx (accessed 27 April 2012).

Oliver, M and Barnes, C (1998) *Disabled People and Social Policy: From exclusion to inclusion.* London: Longman.

Patients Association (2011) *We've Been Listening, Have You Been Learning?* Harrow: Patients Association.

Pattison, S and Wainwright, P (2010) Is the 2008 NMC *Code* ethical? *Nursing Ethics*, 17(1): 9–18.

Pavlish, C, Brown-Saltman, K, Hersh, M, Shirk, M and Rounkle, A (2011) Nursing priorities, actions, and regrets for ethical situations in clinical practice. *Journal of Nursing Scholarship*, 43(4): 385–95.

Payne, M (2000) *Teamwork in Multiprofessional Care.* London: Macmillan.

Perkins, N, Penhale, B, Reid, D, Pinkley, L, Hussein, S and Manthorpe, J (2007) Partnership means protection? Perceptions of the effectiveness of multiagency working and the regulatory framework within adult protection in England and Wales. *Journal of Adult Protection*, 9(3): 19–23.

Phair, L and Heath, H (2010) Neglect of older people in formal care settings part one: new perspectives on definition and the nursing contribution to multiagency safeguarding work. *Journal of Adult Protection*, 12(3): 5–13.

Pinkney, L, Penhale, B, Manthorpe, J, Perkins, N, Reid, D and Hussein, S (2008) Voices from the frontline: social work practitioners' perceptions of multiagency working in adult protection in England and Wales. *Journal of Adult Protection*, 10(4): 12–24.

Pridmore, JA and Gammon, J (2007) A comparative review of clinical governance arrangements in the UK. *British Journal of Nursing*, 16(12): 720–3.

Pring, J (2011) *Longcare Survivors: The biography of a care scandal.* Layerthorpe: Disability News Service.

Pritchard, J (2001) Neglect, in Pritchard, J (ed.) *Good Practice with Vulnerable Adults.* London: Jessica Kingsley, pp225–44.

Pritchard, J (2008) Survivors explain healing through group work, in Pritchard, J (ed.) *Good Practice in Safeguarding Adults.* London: Jessica Kingsley, pp234–57.

Professions Australia (2004) Definition of profession. Available online at www.professions.com.au/define profession.html (accessed 1 May 2012).

Quarmby, K (2008) *Getting Away with Murder: Disabled people's experience of hate crime in the UK.* London: SCOPE.

Reder, P and Duncan, S (2004) Making the most of the Victoria Climbié inquiry. *Child Abuse Review*, 13: 95–114.

Reece, A (2010) Leading the change from adult protection to safeguarding adults: more than just semantics. *Journal of Adult Protection*, 12(3): 30–4.

Robb, B (1967) *Sans Everything.* London: Thomas Nelson.

Roper, N, Logan, W and Tierney, A (1983) *Using a Model for Nursing.* Edinburgh: Churchill Livingstone.

Rowe, MM and Sherlock, H (2005) Stress and verbal abuse in nursing: do burned out nurses eat their young? *Journal of Nursing Management*, 13: 242–8.

Royal College of Nursing (RCN) (2003a) *Defining Nursing.* London: Royal College of Nursing.

Royal College of Nursing (RCN) (2003b) *Clinical Governance: An RCN resource guide.* London: RCN.

Royal College of Nursing (RCN) (2005) *Managing Stress: A guide for nurses.* London: RCN.

Royal College of Nursing (RCN) (2006) *The Impact and Effectiveness of Interprofessional Education in Primary Care: An RCN literature review.* London: RCN.

Royal College of Nursing (RCN) (2011) *Meeting the Health Needs of People with Learning Disabilities: Guidance for nursing staff.* London: RCN.

Royal College of Psychiatrists (RCP) (2004) *The Rowan Report: Implications and advice. Guidance notes for members.* Available online at www.rcpsych.ac.uk/pdf/Rowan.pdf (accessed 15 March 2012).

Ryan, J and Thomas, F (1987) *The Politics of Mental Handicap.* London: Free Association Books.

Sachs-Ericsson, N, Gayman, MD, Kendall-Tackett, K, Lloyd, DA, Medley, A, Collins, N, Corsentino, E and Sawyer, K (2010) The long term impact of childhood abuse on internalizing disorders among older adults: the moderating role of self esteem. *Ageing and Mental Health*, 14(4): 489–501.

Saltvedt, I, Opdahl Mo, ES, Fayers, P, Kaasa, S and Sietvold, O (2002) Reduced mortality in treating acutely sick, frail older patients in a geriatric evaluation and management unit: a prospective randomised trial. *Journal of the American Geriatric Society*, 50(5): 792–8.

Sanders, K and Chaloner, C (2007) Voluntary euthanasia: ethical concepts and definitions, *Nursing Standard*, 21(35): 41–4.

Sandmoe, A and Kirkevold, M (2010) Nurses' clinical assessments of older adults who are suspected victims of abuse: an exploratory study in community care in Norway. *Journal of Clinical Nursing*, 20: 94–102.

Saunders, M (1998) Risk management, in Thompson, T and Mathias, P (eds) *Standards and Learning Disability*, 2nd edition. London: Bailliere Tindall, pp248–60.

Scanlon, A and Lee, GA (2007) The use of the term vulnerability in acute care: why does it differ and what does it mean? *Australian Journal of Advanced Nursing*, 24(3): 54–9.

Schmitt, MH (2001) Collaboration improves the quality of care: methodological challenges and evidence from US health care research. *Journal of Interprofessional Care*, 15(1): 47–66.

Seedhouse, D. (2009) *Ethics: The heart of health care*, 3rd edition. Chichester: Wiley-Blackwell.

Sellman, D (2011) *What Makes a Good Nurse?* London: Jessica Kingsley.

Slettebo, A (2006) Empowerment in nursing homes: lessons for district nursing? *British Journal of Community Nursing*, 11(3): 115–18.

Solum, EM, Slettebo, A and Hauge, S (2008) Prevention of unethical actions in nursing homes. *Nursing Ethics*, 15(4): 536–48.

Stenbock-Hunt, B and Sarvimaki, A (2011) The meaning of vulnerability to nurses caring for older people. *Nursing Ethics*, 18(1): 31–41.

Straughair, C (2011) Safeguarding vulnerable adults: the role of the registered nurse. *Nursing Standard*, 25(45): 49–56.

Tadd, V (1994) Professional codes: an exercise in tokenism? *Nursing Ethics*, 1(11): 15–23.

Taylor, K and Dodd, K (2003) Knowledge and attitudes of staff towards adult protection. *Journal of Adult Protection*, 5(4): 26–32.

Thompson, I, Melia, KM, Boyd, KM and Horsburgh, D (2006) *Nursing Ethics*. Edinburgh: Churchill Livingstone.

Toren, O and Wagner, N (2010) Applying an ethical decision making tool to a nurse management dilemma. *Nursing Ethics*, 17(3): 393–402.

Townsend, P (1962) *The Last Refuge: A survey of residential institutions and homes for the aged in England and Wales.* London: Routledge and Kegan Paul.

Ulivi, G, Reilly, J and Atkinson, JM (2009) Protection or empowerment: mental health service users' views on access and consent for non-therapeutic research. *Journal of Mental Health*, 18(2): 161–8.

Ulrich, CN, Taylor, C, Soeken, K, O'Donnell, P, Farrar, A, Danis, M and Grady, C (2010) Everyday ethics: ethical issues and stress in nursing practice. *Journal of Advanced Nursing*, 66(11): 2510–19.

Walshe, K (2003) *Inquiries: Learning from failure in the NHS?* London: Nuffield Trust. Available online at www.nuffieldtrust.org.uk/ecomm/files/Inquiries_Learning_from_Failure.pdf (accessed 2 May 2011).

Wardhaugh, J and Wilding, P (1998) Towards an explanation of the corruption of care, in Allott, M and Robb, M (eds) *Understanding Health and Social Care: An introductory reader.* London: Sage/Open University Press.

Weaver, K, Morse, J and Mitcham, C (2008) Ethical sensitivity in professional practice: a concept analysis. *Journal of Advanced Nursing*, 62(5): 607–18.

Welsh Government (2012) *Social Services (Wales) Bill: Consultation document.* Cardiff: Welsh Government.

Wheeler, H (2012) *Law, Ethics and Professional Issues for Nursing: A reflective and portfolio-building approach.* London: Routledge.

White, C (2011) Safeguarding against abuse and harm, in Atherton, D and Crickmore, D (eds) *Learning Disabilities: Toward inclusion*, 6th edition. Edinburgh: Churchill Livingstone, pp197–214.

White, C, Holland, E, Marsland, D and Oakes, P (2003) The identification of environments and cultures that promote the abuse of people with intellectual disabilities: a review of the literature. *Journal of Applied Research in Intellectual Disabilities*, 16(1): 1–9.

Whitelock, A (2009) Safeguarding in mental health: towards a rights-based approach. *Journal of Adult Protection*, 11(4): 30–42.

Winterstein, T-B (2012) Nurses' experiences of the encounter with elder neglect. *Journal of Nursing Scholarship*, 441: 55–62.

Women's Aid (2012) Domestic violence statistics. Available online at www.womensaid.org.uk/domestic_violence_topic.asp?section=0001000100220041&sectionTitle=Domestic+violence+%28general%29 (accessed 2 April 2012).

World Health Organization (WHO) (2002) *World Report on Violence and Health.* Geneva: WHO.

World Health Organization (WHO) (2005) Landmark Study on Domestic Violence. Available online at www.who.int/mediacentre/news/releases/2005/pr62/en/index.html (accessed 2 April 2012).

Statutes

Adult Support and Protection (Scotland) Act 2007
Adults with Incapacity (Scotland) Act 2000
Corporate Manslaughter and Corporate Homicide Act 2007
Equality Act 2010
Health and Safety at Work etc. Act 1974
Human Rights Act 1998
Mental Capacity Act 2005
Mental Health Act 1983
Mental Health (Amendment) Act 2007
Public Health Act 1984
Public Health (Infectious Diseases) Regulations 1998
Public Interest Disclosure Act 1998
Road Traffic Act 1998
Sexual Offences Act 2003
Social Services (Wales) Bill 2012
Terrorism Act 2000

Index